Health Humanities in Postgraduate Medical Education

A Handbook to the Heart of Medicine

EDITED BY

Allan D. Peterkin, MD
Professor of Psychiatry and Family
Medicine and Director
Program in Health, Arts, and Humanities
University of Toronto

Anna Skorzewska, MD
Assistant Professor of Psychiatry
University of Toronto

OXFORD
UNIVERSITY PRESS

OXFORD
UNIVERSITY PRESS

Oxford University Press is a department of the University of Oxford. It furthers
the University's objective of excellence in research, scholarship, and education
by publishing worldwide. Oxford is a registered trade mark of Oxford University
Press in the UK and certain other countries.

Published in the United States of America by Oxford University Press
198 Madison Avenue, New York, NY 10016, United States of America.

CIP data is on file at the Library of Congress
ISBN 978–0–19–084990–0

9 8 7 6 5 4 3 2 1

Printed by Webcom Inc., Canada

For Olaf and Katherine, Andreas, Jan, and Sam. (AS)
In memory of Robert Pierre Tomas, a much-loved
renaissance man. (AP)

CONTENTS

Foreword—At the Coalface: Engaging the Humanities in Medical Education

ARNO K. KUMAGAI

Despite (or perhaps because of) the virtual explosion in biomedical knowledge in the past century, there is a growing interest in including the humanities in health professions education. How does one "shoehorn" the humanities—literature, art, theatre, philosophy, history, and the social sciences—into an already overstuffed curriculum, and what is their role in the development of physicians?

One argument for the value of the humanities is that medicine is not a science per se but a social and ethical practice: a practice in which science is applied to the care of human beings in order to alleviate suffering and enhance health. To effectively provide healthcare for individuals during moments of great vulnerability and need, we must understand them in all the complexity of their identities, histories, stories, social relationships, emotions, thoughts, values, and perspectives. This type of knowledge, however, differs greatly from the technical rationality of the biomedical sciences[1] and calls for different types of teaching and learning. The education of physicians in this framework, therefore, becomes a profoundly moral and social undertaking.

In this context, including the humanities in the education of physicians on a postgraduate (residency, fellowship, or junior doctor) level poses several challenges that are different than those encountered when teaching medical students. First, with residents, there is less time for traditional didactic lectures compared to medical school, and there is a constant tension between learning and patient care. Given these competing demands, more learning is done at the "coalface of clinical practice," that is, in clinics and emergency rooms, on the wards, in intensive care units, and in operating rooms. Second, patience runs thin: residents are often tired, stressed out, and constantly distracted by pages, nurses' calls, and patient questions and concerns. They have little freedom to step away in quiet reflection.[2] Third, because opportunities to teach are often dependent on clinical demands and are often directed at learners of widely varying levels, teaching must be "on the fly" and flexible to meet educational needs. Fourth and probably most importantly, teaching and learning about the humanities in the setting of postgraduate training face the challenge of the learners themselves: no longer are they new to medicine; no longer are they moved with a naïve sense of awe and wonder at the sight of human struggles. Instead, steeped in the more deleterious aspects of the so-called "hidden curriculum,"[3] residents may react to such encounters with cold detachment, withdrawal from feeling pain (or empathy), and even a sense of irritation that this "soft stuff" gets in the way of delivering efficient medical care.

There is, however, an advantage to introducing the humanities in the context of postgraduate education. If carefully planned and done well, learners can draw direct connections between core human values and their daily work. They can appreciate "moments of being," in Virginia Woolf's phrase,[4] in which some small occurrence causes resonance deep within the self. They can draw inspiration from the struggles of their patients and turn their attention toward advocacy and social justice. They can open themselves up to the opportunity of forming deeply personal connections with their patients and of bearing witness to the enactment of the deeply humanistic and ethical values of this most human of professions.

The essays contained within this volume explore the ways in which different disciplines within the humanities may be engaged in teaching and learning on a postgraduate level. Among the chapters, there are varying degrees of balance between theoretical perspectives and practical applications—both of which are essential

HEALTH HUMANITIES IN POSTGRADUATE MEDICAL EDUCATION

in effective teaching. Each chapter incorporates a systematic review of existing literature, but this is an emerging area of emphasis in medical education and in many cases published resources are scant. Many of the principles derived from these works are thus general and may be applied to a great variety of training programs; others may be very effective in certain specialties and totally ineffective in others. This variability of approach is not a weakness but a strength: it emphasizes the importance of adapting teaching to context, educational needs, and identities of learners. Resources listed in the Appendix suggest ways of deepening both knowledge and practice.

The essays in this book offer new insights but also provoke a lot of as yet unanswered questions. For instance, how *do* the humanities make better doctors? How is the pedagogy of teaching the humanities different from that of the biomedical and clinical sciences? How can one effectively teach not just in seminars and lectures but in the clinical moment, "at the bedside?" How can we involve patients not just as objects of learning but as agents in this type of teaching? What ways other than narrative medicine can stories be taught and learned? How do we reimagine medical ethics in a social and societal context—that is, looking at ethics through the lens of social justice, critical consciousness,[5] and "structural competency?"[6] How do we design faculty development to effectively teach in these areas? And finally, and very importantly, as discussed in Chapter 10, how do we *assess* such learning?

Answering these questions and the challenges of teaching the humanities on a postgraduate level deserve to be the subject of further conversations. This book, however, represents an excellent start.

References

1. Kumagai AK. From competencies to human interests: ways of knowing and understanding in medical education. *Acad Med.* 2013;89:978–983.

2. Kumagai AK, Naidu T. Reflection, dialogue, and the possibilities of space. *Acad Med.* 2015;90:283–288.

3. Hafferty FW. Beyond curriculum reform: confronting medicine's hidden curriculum. *Acad Med.* 1998;73:403–407.

4. Wear D, Zarconi J, Kumagai A, Cole-Kelly K. Slow medical education. *Acad Med.* 2015;90:289–293.

5. Kumagai AK, Lypson ML. Beyond cultural competence: critical consciousness, social justice, and multicultural education. *Acad Med.* 2009;84:82–87.

6. Metzl JM, Hansen H. Structural competency: theorizing a new medical engagement with stigma and inequality. *Soc Sci Med.* 2014;103:126–133.

Acknowledgments

With thanks to all of our fine authors, to Dr. Sal Spadafora, Vice-Dean Post-MD Education, University of Toronto, for his support of this project; to Dr. Molyn Leszcz and Mount Sinai Hospital for their ongoing support for the humanities in health education; to Marieclaire White for editorial support; and to Prof. Alan Bleakley and our colleagues in the Program in Health, Arts, and Humanities for editorial review and creative suggestions.

Contributors

Shannon Arntfield, MSc, MD, FRSCS
Assistant Professor
Department of Obstetrics and Gynecology
Western University
London Health Sciences Center
London, Ontario, Canada

Susan E. Bélanger
History of Medicine Program
Faculty of Medicine, University of Toronto
Toronto, Ontario, Canada

Carrie Bernard, MD, MPH, CCFP, FCPC
Associate Program Director, Curriculum and Remediation
Department of Family and Community Medicine
University of Toronto
Toronto, Ontario, Canada

Amanda Chen, BSc (Hons)
Faculty of Medicine, University of Toronto
Toronto, Ontario, Canada

Paul Robert D'Alessandro, MD, MSc
Pediatrics Resident
University of British Columbia
Vancouver, British Columbia, Canada

Zac Feilchenfeld, MD, MHPE
Clinical Associate, Division of General Internal Medicine
Sunnybrook Health Sciences Centre
Faculty of Medicine, University of Toronto
Toronto, Ontario, Canada

Farah Friesen, MI
Education Knowledge Broker
    and Program Coordinator
Centre for Faculty
    Development
Faculty of Medicine, University
    of Toronto at Li Ka Shing
    Knowledge Institute
St. Michael's Hospital
Toronto, Ontario, Canada

Lu Gao, MD
Resident in Psychiatry
University of Toronto
Toronto, Ontario, Canada

Neda Ghiam, MD, MHSc
Pediatrician
Toronto, Ontario, Canada

**Karen Gold, BEd, MSW,
PhD, RSW**
Interprofessional
    Education Lead
Women's College Hospital
Affiliated Scientist
Centre for Ambulatory Care
    Education
Toronto, Ontario, Canada

**Mona Gupta, MD, CM, FRCPC,
PhD, CRCHUM**
Centre l'Hospitalier de
    l'Université de Montréal
Associate Professor
Department of Psychiatry
Université de Montréal
Montréal, Québec, Canada

Peggy Hamilton, BSc
Second-year Medical
    Student
University of Winnipeg
Winnipeg, Minnesota

**Philip C. Hébert, MD,
PhD, FCFPC**
Professor Emeritus
Department of Family and
    Community Medicine
Joint Centre for Bioethics
University of Toronto
Toronto, Ontario,
    Canada

**Kathryn Hynes, MD (2019
Candidate)**
Schulich School of Medicine
    and Dentistry
Western University
London, Ontario, Canada

Craig Irvine, PhD
Director of the Masters
    Program in Narrative
    Medicine
Director of Education of
    the Program in Narrative
    Medicine
Columbia University
New York, New York

Martina Kelly, MA, MbBCh, MICGP, FRCGP, CCFP
Associate Professor, Director
  Undergraduate Family
  Medicine
Department of Undergraduate
  Family Medicine
University of Calgary
Calgary, Alberta, Canada

Arno K. Kumagai
Professor and Vice Chair for
  Education
Department of Medicine
F.M. Hill Chair in Humanism
  Education
Women's College Hospital
University of Toronto
Toronto, Ontario, Canada

Ayelet Kuper, MD, DPhil
Scientist and Associate
  Director
Wilson Centre for Research in
  Education
University Health Network
Staff Physician, Division
  of General Internal Medicine
Sunnybrook Health
  Sciences Centre
Associate Professor and
  Co-Lead for Person-Centred
  Care Education
Department of Medicine
Faculty of Medicine, University
  of Toronto
Toronto, Ontario, Canada

Sylvia Langlois, MSc, OT Reg (ON)
Faculty Lead IPE Curriculum
  and Scholarship
Centre for Interprofessional
  Education
Assistant Professor
Occupational Science and
  Occupational Therapy
University of Toronto
Toronto, Ontario, Canada

Suvendrini Lena, MD, MPH, FRCPC, CSCN (EEG)
Staff Neurologist, Geriatric
  Mental Health
Centre for Addiction and
  Mental Health
Clinical Association Centre for
  Headache Women's College
  Hospital
Toronto, Ontario, Canada

Elysse Leonard, BSc, MA
Film Educator in Residence
Health, Arts, and Humanities
  Program
University of Toronto
Toronto, Ontario, Canada

Chryssa McAlister, MD, MHSc, FRCSC
Department of Ophthalmology
  and Vision Sciences
University of Toronto
McMaster University
Kitchener, Ontario, Canada

L. J. Nelles, MFA, PhD (c)
Educator, Geriatric
  Psychiatry
Reitman Centre, Mt. Sinai
  Hospital, Toronto
Voice and Text Teacher,
  Randolph Academy of
  Performing Arts
York University Department of
  Theatre
Toronto, Ontario, Canada

**Allan D. Peterkin, MD,
FCFP, FRCP**
Professor of Psychiatry and
  Family Medicine,
Director, Health, Arts and
  Humanities Program
and UGME/Post-MD Studies
  Humanities Lead,
University of Toronto
Psychiatrist, Mount Sinai
  Hospital
Senior Fellow, Massey College
Toronto, Ontario, Canada

Jeremy Rezmovitz, MD
Family Medicine Sunnybrook
  Health Sciences Centre
Toronto, Ontario, Canada

Edward Shorter, PhD
History of Medicine Program
Faculty of Medicine, University
  of Toronto
Toronto, Ontario, Canada

**Anna Skorzewska, MA,
MD, FRCPC**
Assistant Professor,
  Department of Psychiatry,
Humanism and
  Professionalism Lead Post-
  MD Education,
University of Toronto
Director, Psychiatric Intensive
  Care Unit
University Health Network
Senior Fellow, Massey College
Toronto, Ontario, Canada

Eva-Marie Stern, MA, RP
Art Psychotherapist, Trauma
  Therapy Program
Women's College Hospital
Assistant Professor,
University of Toronto
Toronto, Ontario, Canada

Michael Tau
Centre for Addiction and
  Mental Health
Department of Psychiatry
Toronto, Ontario, Canada

**Robert Pierre Tomas[†], CFRE,
MInstF (Adv. Dip.)**
Principal, Ethical Fundraising
Fundraising Counsel, Canadian
  Association of Health
  Humanities
Toronto, Ontario, Canada

Shelley Wall, AOCAD, MScBMC, PhD, CMI
Assistant Professor, Biomedical
  Communications Program
Institute of Medical Science,
  Faculty of Medicine,
  University of Toronto;
Department of Biology,
  University of Toronto
  Mississauga
Toronto, Ontario, Canada

Cynthia Whitehead, MD, PhD
Scientist and Director, Wilson
  Centre for Research in
  Education
University Health Network
Vice-President Education and
  Practicing Family Physician
  Women's College Hospital
Associate Professor,
  Department of Family and
  Community Medicine
Faculty of Medicine, University
  of Toronto
Toronto, Ontario, Canada

About the Authors

Shannon Arntfield is the director of the Narrative Medicine Initiative at Western University, which seeks to incorporate narrative knowledge as a tool for patient care and reflection as a learning strategy at all stages of medical education and clinical practice. Her work intentionally extends across the undergraduate, postgraduate, and continuing medical education levels, as well as through public engagement and research inquiry.

Susan E. Bélanger's career at the University of Toronto began with undergraduate training in English literature at Victoria College followed by a library science degree and several years' experience as a bibliographic specialist with the *Dictionary of Canadian Biography* before joining the Faculty of Medicine's History of Medicine Program in 1994. Her review of *Phoenix*, Roderick and Sharon Stewart's groundbreaking 2011 biography of Dr. Norman Bethune, appears in *China Review International* (2014). As the program's administrator and research coordinator she is excited by the opportunity to promote the evolving field of medical/health humanities.

Carrie Bernard is the associate program director, Curriculum and Remediation for the Postgraduate Family Medicine program at the University of Toronto. She completed her MPH in 2012 with a focus on global health and more specifically global health ethics. Dr. Bernard is an active member of the Humanitarian Healthcare

Ethics research group and is currently leading an initiative to develop a novel ethics teaching program for postgraduate family and community medicine at the University of Toronto. She has practiced family medicine since 1999 in Brampton, Ontario.

Amanda Chen is a third-year medical student at the University of Toronto. Alongside her studies, Amanda has a special interest in medical education research. She is currently conducting a critical discourse analysis of compassionate care in Canadian undergraduate medical education accreditation standards.

Paul Robert D'Alessandro received his BSc Hons (Distinction) in Life Sciences from Queen's University, and his MSc (Distinction) in Immunology from the University of Oxford. He attended medical school at Dalhousie University in Halifax, Nova Scotia. Paul is an avid performer, who trained and acted professionally prior to medical school, Paul conducts research using verbatim theatre in medical education.

Zac Feilchenfeld is a general internist in Toronto who completed his masters in health professions education at Maastricht University using a research methodology originating in the social sciences to examine a recent development in medical education.

Farah Friesen received her master of information (library and information science) degree from the University of Toronto in 2013. She works to bridge research and programs and encourage effective knowledge sharing that avoids replicating ideas of one-way information flow and focuses on multiway exchanges of information. Farah is pursuing her PhD through the Institute of Medical Science, Faculty of Medicine, University of Toronto. Her research focus is the integration of knowledge and professional identities in clinician-scientists.

Lu Gao is a resident in the Department of Psychiatry at the University of Toronto.

Neda Ghiam is a pediatrician and a graduate of the MHSc program at the Joint Centre for Bioethics, University of Toronto. Her areas of interest in bioethics are the ethics of physician–patient relationship, patient-centered care, and family-centered care as well as education. Her work focuses on educating physicians and patients and, specifically parents in case of pediatric patients, on how best to honor the interests and the autonomy of the whole family from an ethical perspective.

Karen Gold, BEd, MSW, PhD, has worked as a clinical social worker and educator in healthcare for over 20 years. She is the Interprofessional Education Lead at Women's College Hospital and an Affiliated Scientist at the Centre for Ambulatory Care Education. She has a special interest in arts-based inquiry, narrative pedagogy, and collaborative practice.

Mona Gupta is a psychiatrist at the Centre l'Hospitalier de l'Université de Montréal (CHUM) and a clinician-scientist at the CHUM's research institute. She is also associate professor in the Department of Psychiatry at the University of Montréal. Her broad area of academic interest is the intersection of ethics and epistemology in psychiatry. Her research monograph on ethics and evidence-based psychiatry was published by Oxford University Press in 2014. Dr. Gupta is actively engaged in the bioethics community as a member of the editorial committees of *Bioéthique Online* and the *Journal of Ethics and Mental Health* and chair of the RCPSC Bioethics Committee. Dr. Gupta acknowledges, with gratitude, the assistance of Marie-Josée Gibeault in the literature review concerning postgraduate training in psychiatry.

Peggy Hamilton is an actor and a medical student at the University of Manitoba. She places a high value on the role of The Humanities in medicine, and in particular has an interest in how acting and theater can help health professionals develop the skill of empathy. She explores the depths of humanity using theater, and the complexities of the human body in medicine.

Philip C. Hébert is a professor emeritus in the Department of Family and Community Medicine and a member of the Joint Centre for Bioethics at the University of Toronto. In 1983 he received a PhD in philosophy and in 1984 completed medical school at the University of Toronto. He has written a widely used textbook on medical ethics, *Doing Right: A Practical Guide to Ethics for Physicians and Medical Trainees* (3rd ed., Toronto: Oxford University Press, 2014). Dr. Hébert's most recent book is *Good Medicine: The Art of Ethical Care in Canada* (Toronto, Random House, 2016). He is still trying to figure out the best way to teach medical ethics.

Kathryn Hynes is a medical student at Western University, beginning clerkship in 2017–2018. Her interest in narrative medicine began in first year of medical school and was further developed through a research project exploring patient-centered care in an antenatal unit. She hopes to continue to learn more about how narrative medicine may be incorporated both in medical education and her own future clinical practice.

Craig Irvine holds a PhD in philosophy. For more than 15 years, he has been designing and teaching cultural competency, ethics, narrative medicine, and humanities and medicine curricula for residents, medical students, physicians, nurses, social workers, chaplains, dentists, and other health professionals. He has over 20 years of experience researching the history of philosophy, phenomenology, and narrative ethics and over 25 years of experience teaching ethics, humanities, the history of philosophy, logic, and narrative medicine to graduate and undergraduate students. Craig is co-author of *The Principles and Practice of Narrative Medicine* and has published articles in the areas of ethics, residency education, and literature and medicine. He has presented at numerous national and international conferences on these and other topics.

Martina Kelly is a family physician and director of undergraduate family medicine, Cumming School of Medicine, University of Calgary. She completed her master's in education on reflective writing during clerkship. She has taught sociology and film studies to medical students. Her current research explores the role of touch in clinical practice, with a focus on embodied learning, using interpretative phenomenology and drama.

Ayelet Kuper is a scientist and physician whose critical research program explores the relationships among the epistemology of medicine, the history of medical education, and the nature of the medical curriculum. She is currently particularly interested in understanding how to educate healthcare workers for the promotion of equity and social justice.

Sylvia Langlois, MSc, is an assistant professor in the Department of Occupational Science and Occupational Therapy, as well as the Faculty Lead Interprofessional Education Curriculum and Scholarship at the University of Toronto. She has led the development of the Interprofessional Certificate Program in Health, Arts, and Humanities.

Suvendrini Lena is a neurologist at the Centre for Addiction and Mental Health in Toronto and a published playwright. Her play The Enchanted Loom was professionally produced by Cahoots Theatre at the Factory Theatre in Toronto in 2016. She believes that her work as a playwright and watching the actors embody it and bring it to life has changed who she is as a doctor.

Elysse Leonard is a film educator and program coordinator who works at the intersections between film, mental health, and community engagement. She holds an MA in cinema studies from the University of Toronto, with a research focus on illness narratives in classical and postwar international cinemas. Alongside her co-author Michael Tau, Leonard curates the Cinema Medica film series as part of the Health, Arts, and Humanities program at the University of Toronto. She has written video essays for *The Seventh Art*. At the time of publication, Leonard oversees the Toronto

International Film Festival's Reel Comfort program, which brings film screenings and film-craft workshops to mental health programs across Toronto.

Chryssa McAlister practices as a comprehensive ophthalmologist in Kitchener, Ontario. She is a lecturer in the Department of Ophthalmology and Vision Sciences at the University of Toronto and has academic interests in bioethics and medical history. She completed an MHSc at the Joint Centre for Bioethics in Toronto in 2013 and has developed the current postgraduate surgical ophthalmology ethics curriculum at the University of Toronto. She also maintains an academic appointment at McMaster University.

L. J. Nelles is a professional actor and director and has taught acting, voice, and devising in various university and professional theater training programs in Toronto. Her dissertation looks in-depth at some of the ideas in this chapter regarding the use of theater training to encourage embodied practice in healthcare professionals to whom she delivers theater-based workshops. She is also an educator in geriatric psychiatry at the Reitman Centre, Mt. Sinai Hospital, Toronto, and an interning psychotherapist.

Allan D. Peterkin completed residencies in psychiatry and family medicine at McGill University. He is a professor of psychiatry and family medicine at the University of Toronto, where he heads the Program in Health, Arts, and Humanities (www.health-humanities. com) and serves as Humanities Lead for Undergraduate Medical Education and Post-MD studies. Dr Peterkin is the author of 14 books for children and adults, including works on cultural history, human sexuality, physician well-being, narrative-based healthcare, and reflective capacity

Jeremy Rezmovitz is a family doctor at Sunnybrook Health Sciences Centre in Toronto. He has a background in stand- up comedy and attended three months of Humber School of Comedy before leaving for more practical experience.

Edward Shorter earned a PhD in history from Harvard University in 1968, then later took the basic medical science curriculum in medical school. At the University of Toronto, he was first a member of the Department of History, then assumed in 1991 the Jason A. Hannah Chair in the History of Medicine in the Faculty of Medicine, where he is also a member of the Department of Psychiatry. Among his books are *The Making of the Modern Family* (1975), *Doctors and Their Patients: A Social History* (1985; reprint 1991); *From Paralysis to Fatigue: A History of Psychosomatic Illness in the Modern Era* (1992); *A History of Psychiatry* (1997), and *Before Prozac: The Troubled History of Mood Disorders in Psychiatry* (2009). His *Psychosis of Fear: A History of Catatonia*, written in collaboration with Dr. Max Fink, will appear from Oxford University Press in 2018.

Anna Skorzewska is a psychiatrist and an assistant professor at the University of Toronto Faculty of Medicine. She runs a psychiatric intensive care unit and teaches extensively using arts-based methods, in both postgraduate and continuing professional development. She has been the lead in humanism and professionalism at the faculty of medicine post-MD education at the University of Toronto. She started a film-craft program called Reel Comfort for psychiatric inpatients in collaboration with the Toronto International Film Festival. Dr. Skorzewska was the executive producer of an acclaimed documentary film detailing that work called FACELESS, which has screened at festivals including Big Sky.

Eva-Marie Stern is an art psychotherapist and assistant professor in the Department of Psychiatry, University of Toronto, where she supervises residents' psychodynamic psychotherapy training. She teaches interprofessional seminars on using art creation and witnessing as means to understand trauma and its treatment. She is a founder of WRAP (Women Recovering from Abuse Program) and the Trauma Therapy Program at Women's College Hospital.

Michael Tau is a fourth-year psychiatry resident currently training at the University of Toronto. He has co-curated the Cinema Medica film series through the University of Toronto's Department of Psychiatry for the past five years, and, with Elysse Leonard, has presented on cinema and medical education at international conferences.

Robert Pierre Tomas[†], CFRE, MInstF (Adv. Dip.), studied international law in Europe and has worked in broadcasting and philanthropic fundraising in Canada. His work with charities over the past 20 years has focused on youth organizations; chronic illnesses like diabetes, kidney disease, and HIV; and enhancing medical education through arts-based initiatives. He holds an advanced international diploma in fundraising from the University of Plymouth (UK). Robert drowned tragically on holiday on April 1st, 2018.

Shelley Wall is an assistant professor in the University of Toronto's Biomedical Communications graduate program, a certified medical illustrator, and an inaugural illustrator in residence in the Faculty of Medicine, University of Toronto. She teaches a graduate-level course on graphic medicine within the Institute of Medical Sciences and has offered seminars in graphic medicine and illustration as a means of reflection for medical students, interprofessional education classes, and medical practitioners.

Cynthia Whitehead is the director of The Wilson Centre. A critical social scientist, her research program focuses on questioning assumptions that underpin the processes, products, practices, and structures of health professions education. She is currently particularly interested in studying the history of colonial aspects of medical education, in order to move toward decolonized medical education practices both locally and internationally.

Why Are the Health Humanities Relevant (and Vital) in Postgraduate Medical Education?

ANNA SKORZEWSKA AND ALLAN D. PETERKIN

Introduction

A young internist recommends a short YouTube video to her residents made by a young man living with renal failure. She suggests they will learn as much from the film as from her intended lecture on the subject. They talk about his story the next time they meet.

An intern comes home and picks up his violin after a particularly difficult pediatric surgery fraught with complications that proved equally upsetting to the team.

A psychiatry resident meets regularly for coffee with a friend studying architecture. They begin a dialogue on what makes a good, patient-centered hospital.

If you were to ask these physicians what role the arts and humanities played in their working lives, they might answer that they were just doing something they liked. But if you were to press them to tell you what was really happening, you would see that they were creating a space for creative reflection and for thinking and feeling "outside the [medical] box."

These days doctors at all levels of experience are struggling to find meaning in their work in the context of sub-specialization, dwindling resources, low job satisfaction, and burnout.[1,2] As we will see, near-worship at the altar of evidence-based medicine (EBM) has somehow diminished appreciation for the doctor's subjective experience of working with patients. Instinct, intuition, and imagination are difficult to measure and perhaps, for this reason, are not typically seen as "belonging" in the science of medicine. Yet the art of medicine is equally important for good healthcare, especially given the humbling fact that, despite technological advances, we still only manage illness and rarely cure it.

This book fills a significant gap in health humanities education. The medical and health humanities as a discipline have become widespread. There are journals, institutes, and associations worldwide. Throughout undergraduate medical education, new courses, electives, programs, and research are proliferating. Yet there is very little officially documented about relevance and efficacy in postgraduate medical education. This book provides both a rigorous argument for using the arts and humanities in postgraduate medical education and a practical "how-to" that will guide you in developing arts and humanities initiatives in your own program or medical school. Each chapter will provide ideas, hands-on lesson plans, and resources to pave the way forward.

Many senior and respected physician educators argue that medicine has been so reduced to "expert knowledge" and technical skill that it has lost its soul. They feel that the arts and humanities will help put what is missing back into the practice of medicine in order to improve patient care and clinical outcomes.[3–9]

Flexner himself, responsible for imposing rigorous scientific standards in medical education, thought that the "infatuation with the hyper-rational world of German medicine created an excellence in science that was not balanced by a comparable excellence in clinical caring."[10]

Yet, as we will see, there is still strong skepticism about the benefits of arts and humanities in medical education.[11] A key argument is that there are few quantitative studies and very little "hard evidence" to support the claims made. This volume hopes to contribute to the recognition that arts and humanities can play an important role in medical education not only at the postgraduate level (which is the focus here) but at all levels of medical education and practice. We hope that it will inspire the kind of ongoing discourse and inquiry that demonstrate the benefits of our field not only to good clinical outcomes and patient satisfaction but also to physicians themselves and their sense of personal well-being.

The authors contributing to this book have a wealth of experience in the hands-on use of the arts and humanities in medical education. They systematically summarize the experience of others as outlined in the existing literature, then share with you their practical strategies and innovations in their fields of expertise.

Medical Humanities—A Very Short History

The term "medical humanities" was first used by George Sarton in the 1940s in a journal of the history of science, medicine, and civilization.[6,12,13] It was picked up again later in the 1960s in the context of medical education. By the late 1950s, following changes prompted by the Flexner report and the scientific streamlining of medical education, medical educators were beginning to be concerned about the relative importance given to scientific knowledge and inquiry and the devaluing of other aspects of medicine concerned with clinical skills. In 1957 the Case Western Reserve medical school first introduced programming that would incorporate something other than medical knowledge and skill.[13] In 1967 a new medical school at Penn State instituted one of the first programs in medical humanities, a forerunner of subsequent programs.[12] History of medicine as a discipline became more widespread in the 1950s, and the field of bioethics exploded in the 1960s. In 1972, the Institute of Medical Humanities, incorporating a greater breadth of humanities teaching, was founded at the University of Texas at Galveston. By the 1980s, social sciences were also added to teaching curricula to address issues related to philosophical, sociological, and anthropological aspects of medical culture.

There are now dozens of journals devoted to the medical humanities worldwide. In the United States the *Journal of Medical Humanities*, the *Journal of Medicine and Philosophy*, *Literature and Medicine*, and the *Yale Journal for Humanities in Medicine* are prominent examples. In England, *BMJ's Medical Humanities*, *Medical History*, and *Social History of Medicine* are fulfilling that function. Canada's *ARS MEDICA—A Journal of Medicine, the Arts and Humanities*, founded at the University of Toronto, began publishing in 2002.[6,12–14] (See Appendix for a more complete list.)

The medical humanities, now more commonly called the "health humanities" (to be more inclusive of other health professions) have been defined as "an integrated, interdisciplinary, philosophical approach to recording and interpreting human experiences of illness, disability, and medical intervention."[15] The medical humanities are expressly concerned with two areas of healthcare: fostering a deeper understanding of and care for the patient, by emphasizing the human side of medicine, and providing a unique space in which to question, analyze, and critique contemporary practice while encouraging self-reflection among health professionals. There is increasingly a third area with which the medical humanities are concerned, that of physician well-being as linked to reflective capacity.

The health humanities now incorporate several fields, including philosophy, history, the arts (literature/narrative, visual art, drama/theatre, dance, music, and film), anthropology, sociology, and bioethics. (Most of these areas are included as chapter subjects here.)

Although we cannot engage fully with all of the arguments for promoting the health humanities in teaching residents and junior doctors, there are many that are included throughout this book—from the fostering of humility in the face of what medicine cannot do to redressing the high toll that the current practice of medicine takes on physician's well-being. We question the blind faith our profession has placed in the ability of biomedical evidence to guide us and argue passionately for the creation of a safe, vital space for critical and creative reflection that nurtures educators, learners, and practitioners across disciplines.

Reflecting on the Limits of Medical Practice

There are many aspects of medicine that are challenging to our patients, not least that we are rarely able to cure fully but only to mitigate some of the harms brought on by medical illness and suffering. Even then, our remedies, while alleviating some aspects of suffering, bring on their own problems. Sometimes it is unclear whether the disease itself or the remedy is more difficult to live with. "Medical treatments are often over sold and overbought—technical fixes that don't really fix and too often have their own set of harms. . . . For most diseases we have made little progress in the crucial translational step from basic science to clinical practice. We have learned a great deal about how the body works, but much less how to use this knowledge to promote cure."[5]

Diabetes, hypertension, coronary artery disease, arthritis, schizophrenia, epilepsy, inflammatory bowel disease, multiple sclerosis, glaucoma, hypothyroidism—all may be "controlled," but none is cured. These make up the vast majority of the illness burden for our patients, and yet with all our procedures, medications, and technical skills, we have never been able to eradicate these chronic diseases.

As doctors we are sometimes deaf and blind to the very real anguish faced by our patients. If we cannot eliminate the negative effects of our remedies, we could at least provide understanding and solace to our patients who must endure them. Patients come to doctors not only with their ailments but with their deep suffering.

Like all generations of patients before them, they believe that since a physician knows their disease, the physician will also know their suffering. They want ongoing assistance in navigating their illness and in meaning making, something the arts and humanities can nurture in practitioners.

EBM—Successes and Failures

We have been trained to believe, particularly with the advent of EBM, that we need to only look at the "evidence" to know what to do. Few physicians or trainees are encouraged to question critically the wisdom or legitimacy of what they are asked to learn or practice. Yet understanding the limitations of medicine may be very helpful in grounding young doctors.

EBM, with its use of the randomized controlled trial as the gold standard of care, once proclaimed that "a new paradigm for medical practice is emerging. Evidence-based medicine de-emphasizes intuition, unsystematic clinical experience and pathophysiological rationale as sufficient grounds for clinical decision-making and stresses the examination of evidence from clinical research."[16] But in its very design, "social scientists, philosophers, experts in education research, evaluation and measurement and individuals with expertise in studying and understanding the relational and interpretive aspects of individualized patient care" were excluded.[17] Tonelli points to the critical question unanswered by EBM about the usefulness of the role of population-derived evidence in individual care.[18] Population-derived evidence can guide but cannot completely determine clinical decision-making in medicine. In the clinical encounter, there is always an unalienable subjectivity and singularity of experience that comes to bear for both the patient and the doctor.

Even on its own terms, EBM frequently cannot live up to its own standards of empiricism. Patient samples are not fully representative, research time frames are too short, there are inappropriate comparators, and sometimes ethical issues prevent studies from including a control group. Negative findings are rarely published, and research funding remains politically and economically driven. Thus, the claims that are made in the name of EBM are often flawed even in a domain that lends itself well to its own methodology!

To require reductionist and positivist types of evidence, as exemplified by EBM, from educational strategies now employed in the health humanities seems misguided and perverse. Many have challenged EBM on epistemological and other philosophical grounds.[15,18,19] Philosophy of science calls into question much of our reductionist understanding of "truth" in science. Even the great philosopher of science, Willard van Orman Quine, himself an empiricist, argued that scientific theory is underdetermined by evidence because the evidence is never sufficient to determine the accuracy of the theory that it purports to explains.[20]

EBM and the Health Humanities— Uneasy Bedmates

An entire book could be devoted to an examination of EBM-based criticisms leveled at the health humanities and the claims upon which these criticisms are based. This is not the purpose of this book. Nevertheless, with funding limitations and time both at a premium in medical education, we cannot simply dismiss these criticisms. While we hope that this book will review and provide some answers, we also must take issue with the kinds of evidence the arts and humanities are called upon to provide. It is certainly true that, if the arbiter of evidence is exclusively quantitative, empirical, and reductionist, the health humanities (and the humanities within the academy at large) have not provided evidence of that kind. Yet, it is still unclear what help or relevance such evidence would actually bring to the table. How do we measure constructs like empathy, moral distress, cultural sensitivity, imaginative capacity, critical thinking, narrative competence, intersubjectivity, and human caring without robbing them of richness, depth, and complexity?

A single example, the much-referenced meta-analysis by Ousager and Johannessen was a subject of close textual analysis by Catherine Belling. She criticizes that review's purported "proof" that only 9 out of 245 papers included in the study provided empirical evidence that humanities curricula in undergraduate medical education had a practical or useful impact on future physicians. In a related critique, Rita Charon points out the flaws in the authors' search engine choice (Medline only) for the studies included in the meta-analysis, their categorization, and even their actual examination (often using abstracts only), thus making it impossible to draw valid conclusions.[21] Belling found that the conclusions might support this assertion if simply quantifying all of the data. Yet examining their data for deeper meaning often revealed the opposite of what the Ousager and Johannesen had claimed. In short Ousager and Johannessen, in analyzing the data, using their "blunt instrument" of measurement missed irony altogether and failed to account for it in their evaluation.[22]

A more interesting question to ask is: What is the value of the arts and humanities in medicine? Asking about value places a different onus on those arguing for their place within medicine. It speaks to the importance we place as human beings on the arts and humanities in society as a whole and asks what this larger debate brings to bear in contexts of healing.

The arts and humanities are not only called on to prove "outcomes" in medicine, but in an age where the marketplace is the arbiter of "value," there has been great pressure to justify their worth within the university and in society as a whole. Helen Small identifies five historical arguments for the humanities and their value as a public good, traces their evolution, and examines their weight in contemporary society. She argues that the humanities have a distinct disciplinary character focusing on the interpretation and evaluation of our culture that takes as its premise the very subjectivity that is absent in many of the sciences and social sciences. She argues for the utility of a discourse that puts pressure on governments and economies about assumptions of merit. (See also Bill Readings' *The University in Ruins* and Kurt Spellmeyer's "Saving the Social Imagination.")[23,24] She argues that the humanities include another kind of discourse that looks at what notions of happiness are and what we collectively really value as human beings.[20] All of these speak equally to some aspect of medicine.

Perhaps Jonathan Bates puts it most succinctly when saying that "research in the humanities is the only activity that can establish the meaning of such a question." He adds moreover that it is the only activity that can ask with some impertinence: "What is the value of research in the sciences?"

In other words, the arts and humanities in different ways create a space for healthy skepticism and questioning, for examining our culture, and for honing critical and moral reflection.[25] If an unexamined life is not worth living, what of an unexamined medical life?

Humanities scholars have different methods and tools within their fields—in science it is most often statistics and quantifiable data. In history, sociology, and anthropology it is empirical investigation, interpretation, and close analysis of texts using deductive reasoning. In philosophy and literary studies, it is analytical thinking, close reading, and reason. These tools must be seen as just as legitimate in the field of medical humanities (and medicine at large) as they are in the university history course or the philosophy seminar.

The sheer range of knowledge acquisition now required in medicine has become so overwhelming that we have forgotten to ask ourselves if our current methodologies even make sense, if our patterns of care are truly effective, and if we are taking caring of ourselves and of our patients seriously enough. Each of the chapter authors in this book believe passionately that the health humanities help in the infinitely difficult task of translating what we know (provisionally) into what we should do in order to help and not harm (empirically). Science (and EBM) alone cannot give us the answers.

How the Humanities Assist Residents in Identity Formation, Meaning Making, and Self-Care

Training physicians have less control over their lives than their supervisors.[1,26] Many of the problems faced by residents, junior doctors, and fellows in their education revolve around issues that do not even get named or discussed. These include the impact of physician encounters on patients and the important role of noncognitive attributes in future healers, including exploring feelings as a part of learning and tolerating ambiguity and uncertainty. High levels of responsibility, intense contact with people, time restrictions, role uncertainty, sleep deprivation, and social isolation are linked to stress in any profession but perhaps particularly in medicine. In postgraduate training, residents must deal directly and responsibly with suffering, fear, death, ambiguity, and problem patients and staff. They are also busy surviving, worried about making mistakes, trying to please.[26]

How then to arrive at a balance of knowledge and skill with the ability to communicate, understand, and consider the patient as a unique human being situated in the world by culture, gender, social status, and personal beliefs? And how can doctors do this while taking care of themselves and avoiding burnout? Each of the chapters that follows convincingly makes the argument that the arts and humanities hold the key.

In our view, the health humanities incorporate ways of thinking to complement content-based knowledge and practice-based skills. As you will see throughout this book, they can help trainees develop critical thinking (the ability to question, analyze, and evaluate information to form a judgment). They help foster narrative competence—the ability to work with stories, to listen optimally, and to co-construct the meaning of illness and healing with patients over time. They foster the ability to *see*—both literally and metaphorically—and to *reflect*—to step back and learn from past experience so that it can be applied in the here and now. They promote the ability for self-care by helping the resident explore the following questions about themselves:

Who am I? (As a person with assumptions, insights, biases, and personal values)

What Am I? (What does it mean to be a doctor in a postmodern, highly technological world?)

Where am I? (What sociocultural and economic factors shape how I provide care to my patients, their families and communities?)

How do the answers to these questions affect how I do my work?

and about their patients:

Who is my patient? (What kind of person is my patient? What are his or her values? What are his or her beliefs?)

What is my patient's cultural and social background?

Where is my patient? (How does my patient live? How does he or she see the hospital, the clinic office?)

How do the answers to these questions affect my clinical decisions?

The State of the Art(s) in Medicine

For some time now, in the United States, the United Kingdom, and Canada, the inclusion of programs in the medical humanities as well as mandatory humanities curricula in undergraduate medical education has become widespread. (For example, a recent survey of all 17 Canadian medical schools conducted in 2016 by Peterkin, Brett-MacLean, Kidd, and Beausoleil confirmed the presence of such teaching in *all* undergraduate programs.) The offerings by medical/health humanities divisions in medical schools in North America and the United Kingdom are currently rich and diverse. They include watching films, learning to interpret paintings, performing close readings of literary texts, and reflective and creative writing.

They can also include personal reflective portfolios, seminars about the interface between the arts and medicine, and the arts for health movement. Quite excitingly, they often invite trainees to develop an artistic practice themselves, which can afford new forms of creative expression and reflection but also encourage learning with *both* sides of the brain. They honor thoughts and feelings, the subjective and the objective. These endeavors can help reduce the gap between biomedicine and the human sciences, such as philosophy, history, sociology, and anthropology. They can facilitate interdisciplinary and interprofessional teaching and research, model a patient-centered approach to medical care, challenge biomedical arrogance, and equip doctors to meet the moral challenges of practice not covered expressly (or adeptly) by medical education.

Sadly, such initiatives fall off in many residency programs when they are most needed. (Reasons for this are discussed later.) The humanities can help counteract burnout and cynicism which we know increase during residency training (in conjunction with declining empathy levels[27]). Reflective, creative practitioners take better care of their patients, but they also take better care of themselves, because they have new tools to challenge their assumptions and to sustain their personal values and sense of purpose while providing optimal care.

Recently, in both Canada and the United States, there has been a shift to competency-based models of medical education.[28] Of the seven competencies described in the current Canadian CanMeds model, for example, a majority have to do with the so-called soft, non-scholarly skills of medicine including communication, collaboration, professionalism, advocacy, and leadership.[28] Interestingly, although these competencies comprise five of the seven, only a very small percentage of explicit curricular time is currently devoted to them, with formal training remaining largely dedicated to the "medical expert" and the scholarly competencies. This is in part due to the difficult task of determining how to teach these competencies which are not so much "soft" as complex and difficult to teach. More sophisticated educational approaches are clearly needed rather than the simple transmission of knowledge and skill.

Rita Charon in her commentary on the contribution of the humanities in medical practice asks: "Who are the students?" a question she finds both salient and missing. She answers, "all clinicians," finding room and reason to include clinical learners at all levels of training and practice.[21]

In this book we address postgraduate medical training and argue that it is perhaps an even better place to include medical humanities education. As William Carlos Williams has said, "it takes time to become a doctor." Medical students are busy mastering the basic tools of medicine: both the knowledge and the skills. Gaining this mastery is stressful enough, and complexity and nuance can only be grappled with once the basics are in place. Once these are "mastered" and trainees move on to postgraduate training, they enter a world in which they have much more independence and autonomy. It is at this moment that all of the uncertainty, the gray areas and murkiness in medicine, emerge. It is here that generalities, laws, rules, and norms are helpful but insufficient to make thoughtful and timely decisions. It is here that understanding cultural differences, a patient's individual situation, and the beliefs and values of patients must be incorporated into decisions in the care plan.

Curricula, Hidden and Otherwise

Few residents and other medical trainees are encouraged to question the wisdom or legitimacy of what they are asked to learn or to reflect on their experience of power and hierarchy in their training. Curricula are (after all) designed by senior faculty and overseen by licensing bodies, specialty organizations, colleges and institutions, and they provide "standards of practice." Most of us refer to "The (official) Curriculum" as the formal, stated, and intended body of knowledge we are all meant to master. This is the actual course of study and consists of teaching, evaluation of teaching methods, syllabi, and other material used in any educational setting from lecture halls to labs, to seminar rooms, the bedside, and clinics. The Informal (or delivered) Curriculum is "what actually happens." As Delese Wear reminds us, it consists of "idiosyncratic, popup, and often unplanned instruction that takes place between anyone who is teaching (attendings, residents, or other healthcare professionals) and trainees. It reflects what teachers believe trainees should acquire in terms of knowledge, skills, values, and attitudes."[29]

The Hidden Curriculum, in contrast, involves what is taught inadvertently and usually has a negative connotation. This concept originally comes from the educational rather than the medical literature, and it contains messages both ideological and subliminal from the formal and informal curricula. The hidden curriculum is transmitted through individuals through looks, gestures, tone, and behaviors but also through the structures and practices of institutions, including hospitals and universities. Dr. Fred Hafferty, who first applied notions of the Hidden Curriculum to medicine, described it as "understandings, customs, rituals, and taken-for-granted aspects of what goes on in the life-space we call medical education."[30] It thus consists of unexamined practices, messages, assumptions, values, rules, protocols, privileges, use of language, manifestations of power and domination, indifference to inequity, and prioritization of what is important and less important in the knowledge to be transmitted.

Residents often have trouble defining the Hidden Curriculum, but they generally do not have difficulty identifying it when they encounter it. The Hidden Curriculum manifests through negative role modeling and unprofessional behavior from preceptors and supervisors. In the face of the Hidden Curriculum, learners feel discomfort because they receive mixed messages, and they may feel silenced or powerless in the face of unprofessional or even harmful behaviors.

Medical students generally enter medical school with greater empathy, compassion, and idealism than when they leave it. This trend continues in residency. As we will see, the humanities provide a critical framework for fostering the sophistication required to deal with such difficult educational goals as unpacking power differentials and identifying and understanding mixed messages that are delivered in the Hidden Curriculum. It is often more fruitful to discuss a visual or literary text in all its richness and depth than to point fingers within a team or at a powerful senior faculty member.

Delese Wear has described the contributions of the medical/ health humanities in relation to the development of self and sensibility as learners "move through an increasingly complex life in medicine, examining themselves, their patients, their profession, and the culture in which they serve."[29] Simply put, the humanities help residents and practitioners to think, empathize, argue, evaluate, and express themselves—all essential qualities in a clinical life.

This Book: A Guide and an Invitation

This volume serves as a handbook on the use of the arts and humanities in postgraduate medical education—a field yet to be fully tapped and waiting to flourish. You may be a resident leader or an educator. Feel free to start with chapters/themes that interest you most. Try out the suggested lesson plans and then develop your own, based on the learning needs of residents in your program.

Authors are from multiple clinical and academic disciplines and convey the richness of an interprofessional, multidisciplinary approach. Each chapter provides a thorough literature review as well as some theoretical arguments for the area under consideration. (This will be helpful as you make a case for creating new learning opportunities to the chief of your department.)

Each chapter (including this one) also provides very practical guidance on implementing new programming and includes actual sample lesson plans and lists of resources for networking and deepening your knowledge. In this way, after reading the book, you will not only have a sense of the existing literature in the area of interest but you will also be able to frame a theoretical argument for its value, use a lesson plan, or create your own research questions using the resources provided. The chapters go back and forth between the social sciences/humanities and the arts, illuminating what each domain has to offer and how the reader might use both the scholarship and the practical suggestions for teaching. Throughout, you will also see how the arts can be healing not only for patients but for the residents themselves.

Elysse Leonard and Michael Tau are also concerned with the "visible," in this case through the lens of a camera, a medium particularly engaging to residents, many of whom who are highly visual learners. They show how film, a narrative, multisensory, durational, and embodied medium, can go beyond the illustrative and instrumental use of moving image culture toward its incorporation as a medium of critical discourse and introspection.

Shannon Arntfield explores the use of narrative medicine, an area which has grown significantly since the early 2000s and perhaps the only arts/humanities curriculum which has gained solid purchase thus far in medical education.[31] She demonstrates how the arts and humanities, in this instance narrative medicine, can highlight interesting paradoxes in medicine while honoring the uniqueness of the story that each patient brings to the clinical setting. (A description of an actual narrative medicine session is provided by Craig Irvine in his Afterword.)

Philip Hebert and his co-authors trace the history of bioethics education in medicine, briefly outlining for us the various philosophical approaches to ethical problems in medicine and the influence of "duty-based" versus "consequentialist" approaches to medical ethics. They include several useful tools to help guide you in ethical dilemmas and decision-making. Ultimately they point out that the role of ethics in medicine is not necessarily to come up with the right answer but to foster a reflective approach to the uncertainties in medicine.

Eva Marie Stern and Shelley Wall explore the visible curriculum, one that will not only improve skills in "seeing" the patient but also help shed light on the Hidden Curriculum (that which is "unseen"). They demonstrate that art can be used as a method of questioning and transforming. They emphasize not only visual art's ability to increase skills in observation but also the benefits of "art-making" (arts-based practice), something a little less common in the existing visual arts and medical education literature.

Zac Feilchenfeld and colleagues provide a very thorough literature review on the use of social sciences in postgraduate medical education as well as a theoretical model for teaching it. Much of their review and suggestions take into consideration the dominant competency framework that now exists in both the United States and Canada, but what they provide extends beyond this current trend in medical education.

L. J. Nelles and colleagues admirably demonstrate through their chapter on theater that medicine is actually an embodied practice. Not only do we "manage" the bodies of our patients but we, ourselves, should seek to be mindful and fully embodied. Theater allows a nonjudgmental forum for exploring many of the difficult themes and uncertainties that we inevitably find in our daily struggles and those of our patients in managing their illnesses and suffering.

Sylvia Langlois and Karen Gold turn to the arts and humanities to foster truly interprofessional dialogue, teamwork, and problem-solving. They underline the relational aspect of medical care not only between healthcare provider and patient but among healthcare providers as team members seeking to provide truly good care.

Edward Shorter and Sue Bélanger share a highly personal overview of the relevance of teaching medical history to residents— emphasizing humility in the face of the provisional nature of medical knowledge at any given moment. History of medicine not only teaches us about lessons from the past but can inspire us in looking to the future.

In response to the longstanding evaluation and legitimacy quandary summarized here, Martina Kelly gives a wonderful overview of the interesting and exciting new ways of capturing, through new research methodologies, the complexity and depth in arts and humanities education that we so desperately need—and not the round peg–square hole accommodation to the quantitative demands of biomedical research but methods that honor the way we construct knowledge in the health humanities and social sciences. To develop the health humanities in postgraduate medicine, we will need to aim for excellence—an excellence with its own aesthetic, relevant to our unique field of study.

Finally, philanthropy expert Robert Pierre Tomas, guides the reader, in his own very personal voice, through the often-frustrating attempts to get funding for innovative, "out of the box" programs within medicine. He provides an overarching vision, from practical tips on how to fund pizza for a medical film series to ways of pursuing the elusive major gift that will solidify a formal program.

Conclusion

The arts and humanities are uniquely positioned to help us all step outside the biomedical arena and turn an engaged, critical gaze on the many practices of medicine. Our trainees need to be given the tools necessary to decipher the arguments made in favor of current research and treatment decisions and to navigate hospital protocols, hierarchies, and values of caring. They need a grounding which will allow them to accompany patients in the face of uncertainty and suffering. We need to nurture our residents to remain curious about the other (and themselves) and to find solace, purpose, and replenishment as they do their work.

If the arts and humanities do no more than make young doctors feel and think more deeply, we will have helped them enormously.

A sample curriculum to accompany this chapter can be found online at http://cahh.ca/resources/ouplesson-plans/.

References

1. Peterkin A. Medical humanities for what ails us. *CMAJ.* 2008;178(5):648.

2. Shanafelt TD, Dyrbye LN, West CP. Addressing physician burnout: The way forward. *JAMA*. 2017;317(9):901–902.

3. Alpert JS, Coles R. Premedical education: A modest proposal repeated. *Arch Intern Med*. 1987;147(4):633–634.

4. Frey JJ 3rd. How the humanities inform medicine. *WMJ*. 2010;109(6):309.

5. Frances A. Putting humanity and the humanities back into medicine (Editorial). *The Huffington Post*. July 30, 2015.

6. Hurwitz B, Dakin P. Welcome developments in UK medical humanities. *J R Soc Med*. 2009;102(3):84–85.

7. Gillon R. Welcome to medical humanities—and why. *J Med Ethics*. 2000;26(3):155–156.

8. Watkins P. Understanding illness and medical humanities. *Clin Med*. 2001;1(2):93.

9. Coles R. The humanities in postgraduate training. *JAMA*. 1987;257(12):1644.

10. Duffy TP. The Flexner report—100 years later. *Yale J Biol Med*. 2011;84(3):269–276.

11. Ousager J, Johannessen H. Humanities in undergraduate medical education: A literature review. *Acad Med*. 2010;85(6):988–998.

12. Hurwitz B. Medical humanities: Lineage, excursionary sketch and rationale. *J Med Ethics*. 2013;39(11):672–674.

13. Cook HJ. Borderlands: A historian's perspective on medical humanities in the US and the UK. *Med Humanit*. 2010;36(1):3–4.

14. Cooke M, Irby DM, Sullivan W, Ludmerer KM. American medical education 100 years after the Flexner report. *N Engl J Med*. 2006;355(13):1339–1344.

15. Evans M. Reflections on the humanities in medical education. *Med Educ*. 2002;36(6):508–513.

16. Evidence-Based Medicine Working Group. Evidence-based medicine: A new approach to teaching the practice of medicine. *JAMA*. 1992;268(17):2420–2425.

17. Wyer PC, Silva SA. Where is the wisdom? I—A conceptual history of evidence-based medicine. *J Eval Clin Pract*. 2009;15(6):891–898.

18. Silva SA, Wyer PC. Where is the wisdom? II—Evidence-based medicine and the epistemological crisis in clinical medicine. Exposition and commentary on Djulbegovic, B., Guyatt, G. H. & Ashcroft, R. E. (2009) *Cancer Control*, 16, 158–168. *J Eval Clin Pract*. 2009;15(6):899–906.

19. Goldenberg MJ. On evidence and evidence-based medicine: Lessons from the philosophy of science. *Soc Sci Med.* 2006;62(11):2621–2632.

20. Quine WV. *Word and Object.* Cambridge, MA: MIT Press; 1960.

21. Charon R. Commentary: Calculating the contributions of humanities to medical practice—Motives, methods, and metrics. *Acad Med.* 2010;85(6):935–937.

22. Belling C. Commentary: Sharper instruments: On defending the humanities in undergraduate medical education. *Acad Med.* 2010;85(6):938–940.

23. Spellmeyer K. Saving the social imaginiation: The function of the humanities at the present time. *College English.* 2012;74(6):567–587.

24. Readings B. *The University in Ruins.* Cambridge, MA: Harvard University Press; 1996.

25. Bate J. *The Public Value of the Humanities.* London: Bloomsbury Academic; 2011.

26. Peterkin AD. *Staying Human During Residency Training: How to Survive and Thrive After Medical School.* 6th ed. Toronto; Buffalo; London: University of Toronto Press; 2016.

27. Neumann M. Empathy decline and its reasons: A systematic review of studies with medical students and residents. *Acad Med.* 2011;86(8):996–1009.

28. Canada RCoPaSo. CanMeds Physician Competency framework. 2016. http://canmeds.royalcollege.ca/en/framework.

29. Wear D, Skillicorn J. Hidden in plain sight: The formal, informal, and hidden curricula of a psychiatry clerkship. *Acad Med.* 2009;84(4):451–458.

30. Hafferty FW, Franks R. The hidden curriculum, ethics teaching, and the structure of medical education. *Acad Med.* 1994;69(11):861–871.

31. Charon R, DasGupta S. Narrative medicine, or a sense of story. *Lit Med.* 2011;29(2):vii–xiii.

2

Redirecting the Clinical Gaze

Film as a Tool of Critical Reflection in Residency Training

ELYSSE LEONARD AND MICHAEL TAU

Introduction

The use of film in medical education dates back at least as far as 1897, when John Macintyre, an ENT surgeon, presented an animated sequence of x-ray images of a knee joint moving at a medical lecture. Many subsequent early films depicted surgical techniques and were intended to be used as a teaching aid for trainees. Since then, film has been used in many different contexts to teach healthcare trainees from various disciplines, increasingly so over the last quarter of the 20th century and into the 21st. Several books have been written about the use of commercial film in medical education, including *Movies & Mental Illness: Using Films to Understand Psychopathology*,[1] *Signs of Life: Cinema & Medicine*,[2] *The Picture of Health: Medical Ethics and the Movies*,[3] and *Cinemeducation: Using Film and Other Visual Media in Graduate and Medical Education*.[4] There is even a peer-reviewed journal dedicated to the intersection of cinema and medicine, *The Journal of Medicine and Movies*. While the second volume of *Cinemeducation* encompasses postgraduate medical education, much of the published literature focuses on the use of film to illustrate concepts, scenarios, or technical skills in the undergraduate setting.

The postgraduate context affords educators an opportunity to move beyond the illustrative and instrumental use of moving image culture toward its incorporation as a medium of critical discourse and introspection. In the transition from undergraduate to postgraduate medical education, learners also undergo an experiential shift in focus from the acquisition of broad information to the deep mastery that results from specialization and clinical practice. With this sense of self-efficacy and competence comes an enriched ethical understanding of the larger health systems within which students operate as well as a heightened awareness of any gaps in their own knowledge and expertise. As a result, the increase in capacity one experiences in residency may be met with an equal increase in feelings of uncertainty and one's own perceived limitations.

Film—a narrative, multisensory, durational, and embodied medium—is well suited to help postgraduate students negotiate the complexities of their identities as healthcare providers, their relationship to clients/patients, and the affective and ethical consequences arising from clinical practice. In advocating for film's utility in teaching medical ethics, Stephen Crawford and Henri Colt cite the dissimilarity of this approach from that of standard medical education as the very source of its efficacy in facilitating higher-order thinking: "[T]hose step-by-step approaches necessarily seek answers, perhaps even one answer, to a particular dilemma, whereas a film strives to fling open doors to multiple questions and may never fully resolve an issue."[3] By asking viewers to participate on an intellectual, emotional, and physical level, the authors argue, film offers students multiple entry points from which to contemplate and discuss topics that may prove paradoxical or otherwise difficult to comprehend. Deep engagement with film texts, which requires close, active observation on the part of the viewer, can prompt residents to not only incorporate the learning of the medical establishment but also to interrogate the very systems that produce and reinforce that learning.

Following a review of the literature on film's various applications in medical education and a discussion of some characteristics of the medium that are conducive to reflection, empathy, and other humanistic experiences, this chapter will outline an alternative approach that privileges discovery, confrontation, and comfort with not-knowing above traditional learning. This model is inspired by the authors' longstanding collaboration on a screening series that invites interdisciplinary scholars and practitioners to explore healthcare topics through the close reading and discussion of film texts. Given the limitations on space, this will by no means be an exhaustive survey of the field; rather, it will offer insight into a specific programming approach and philosophy, one informed by medical and humanities perspectives, as well as pertinent themes and questions that emerge in the discourse. By modeling a close reading of a narrative film, the authors hope to provide educators with a theoretical framework that can be extended to support a wide variety of learning objectives. The books indicated earlier include comprehensive, targeted programming guides and should be considered in conversation with this chapter.

Film in Medical Education: A Review of the Literature

There have been a few relevant reviews covering the nexus of film and medical education, though these are not specific to residency training, as the majority of examples cited relate to teaching medical students or to educating trainees generally. One systematic review examines the body of literature from many dimensions, including specific films used, target audience, chronology, and whether feedback was solicited from participants.[5] A more recent review identified several major themes in the literature and included television shows alongside film: breaking bad news, professionalism, ethics, empathy, doctor-patient communication, cultural competence, managing severe or terminal disease, death and dying, and alcohol or other drugs.[6] These themes reflect an emphasis on the so-called "soft skills" of medicine. For example, many authors locate film's educational impact in its unprecedented ability to cultivate empathy by way of eliciting emotional responses in learners. The "best movies," Crawford and Colt write, "provide us with a vision of reality . . . that strikes the core of our emotional selves and often causes us to think beyond our standard responses to consider alternative ideas." Educators can leverage this affective quality, they argue, to support the development of a range of "emotional and interpretive" skills alongside a range of "rational and analytic" skills. The review by Law et al. also noted that a majority of the publications were focused on psychiatry and mental health, which might be due to the perception of medical teachers and trainees that soft skills are more germane to the culture of mental health relative to other clinical disciplines.[6] Film theory, too, has a legacy of conceptualizing film as analogous to the human mind, mapping certain technical processes onto cognitive processes like attention and memory.[7] For example, a flashback denotes an episodic memory; a close-up is often used to convey enhanced focus. Since residents are often tasked with reconciling seemingly disparate information and experiences, it might be productive to shed the binaries of soft/hard and emotional/rational—and the related binaries of accurate/inaccurate, mind/body—in favor of a more holistic approach that addresses the complex interplay of these qualities within the student-practitioner and within film.

In terms of methodology, a closer examination of the literature reveals a diverse range of approaches to integrating film into medical education. Authors may use entire feature-length films or isolated excerpts. Film-based learning has been variously integrated into existing mandatory lectures or rounds presentations, assigned as obligatory, self-directed learning, and presented as part of elective seminar series or casual "movie clubs." Screenings are often followed by a discussion for trainees to reflect on and integrate knowledge; in some cases, this component is didactic and structured, whereas other models utilize a more open-ended and learner-driven approach. The initiatives described in these articles have been written by authors in North America, Europe, South America, Australia, and Asia.[5]

In line with the film/mind comparison, most residency-specific articles pertain to the field of psychiatry, with select others discussing film as a tool for teaching family medicine residents, internal medicine residents, and surgical residents. A 1979 report on a film discussion group in a psychiatry residency program is often cited as the first article that describes using professional motion pictures to teach medical trainees.[8]

Films as Content-Based Teaching Aids in Residency

Film is often cited as a useful tool for developing psychiatric diagnostic skills.[9-11] The book *Movies & Mental Illness*, now in its fourth edition, is perhaps the most comprehensive example of this approach, providing a sample syllabus that pairs various commercially available movies with proposed diagnoses and extrapolated case histories for fictional characters. An article by Kalra[12] compiles a similar list of films and accompanying diagnoses in describing a voluntary film club for psychiatry residents. This method, a sort of formalized "armchair diagnosis," asks trainees to compare the character(s) represented in each film against their own experience with and knowledge of psychiatric presentations and diagnostic criteria. Hopkins et al. created a five-session seminar series using clips from mainstream films, with residents assigned each as a clinical case and asked to generate a differential diagnosis and treatment options.[13] Within the context of undergraduate medical education, film has been used to teach content about HIV,[14] clinical pharmacology,[15] substance toxidromes and withdrawal syndromes,[16] addiction,[17] and medical microbiology.[18] One reported downside to this content-based approach is that many movies portray psychiatric signs and symptoms in a way that does not correspond with the psychiatric literature or traditional clinical experience.[12] Much of the literature seems to conflate a film's quality and usefulness with its "accuracy," revealing an underlying faith in film's ability to capture reality and reaffirming the institutional values of truth and mastery. If film holds up a mirror to society, however, the image returned is mediated by various political, economic, and aesthetic forces. A more holistic approach to film-based learning is needed to create a space for critical reflection and change, one that acknowledges that film both documents indexical reality and offers a stylized lens through which to interpret it.

Film as a Way of Teaching Psychosocial Dimensions of Medicine

Beyond medical expertise, film has also been used to engage residents' humanistic side and expose them to diverse lifestyles.[19] A neurosurgical residency program implemented a mandatory film and book club to address communication skills, professionalism, and healthcare systems.[20] One author used *The Breakfast Club* (1985) to teach residents about adolescent development and the practice of psychotherapy with teenagers.[21] Clips from the films *The Lost Weekend* (1945) and *When a Man Loves a Woman* (1994) have been used to teach family medicine residents about the role of the family in alcohol use disorders.[22] Excerpts from the television program *ER* have been used to teach medical students psychotherapeutic techniques, including treating patients with personality disorders and breaking bad news.[23] Authors have also devoted articles to film education and end-of-life issues and bereavement,[24] often in the context of fostering clinical communication skills.[25]

Values-Based Learning Objectives

Kalra screened the film *Gothika* (2003) during a voluntary, after-clinic film club for psychiatry residents to spur reflection and discussion about stigma.[26] Another report recommends several films to teach cultural competence in medical students and residents, providing multiple examples of films stratified by ethnicity.[27] There is an extensive body of research devoted to the use of film in teaching medical ethics and professionalism at the undergraduate level.[28,29]

One integrative paper explores several themes in medical education, describing the use of several film clips to teach residents about each of the core competencies defined by the Accreditation Council for Graduate Medical Education. These competencies, which mirror those described in CanMEDS roles used in Canadian and European training, include a combination of expertise- and value-based goals, namely patient care, medical knowledge, practice-based learning and improvement, communication skills, professionalism, and systems-based practice. In this model, screenings are partitioned into modules in which clips are shown, and then prepared discussion questions guide residents toward reflection upon content within each objective.[19]

Impact Measurement

Articles that investigate specific outcomes of film-based learning tend to restrict their focus to qualitative measures such as trainee satisfaction or change in knowledge or attitudes, as assessed by self-report tools. According to a rigorous review, such surveys generally yielded positive results,[6] although, at times, the results were nonsignificant.[20] Matthew Alexander, one of the editors of *Cinemeducation*, notes that the challenges associated with demonstrating the efficacy of film-based learning are shared by the broader field of medical humanities. Most studies are limited by small sample sizes and fail to demonstrate quantifiable, objective changes in student-practitioners. The imperative to demonstrate impact is directly tied to funding sources and the sustainability of arts-based programming, but it presents a dilemma: how does one measure and support exploratory learning, which invites participants to think beyond traditional frames of reference, using methodology that is imbricated in the very systems participants are to exceed? This is a challenge arts-based educators will continue to negotiate as this field expands.

Results of Our Call for Information

In preparing this chapter, the authors put out a call through an international medical humanities listserv to solicit information from healthcare educators implementing film in their practice. The breadth of responses serves as a testament to the malleability of the cinematic medium as an educational tool. One physician described a series of self-produced short films, created in collaboration with a colleague, to accompany specific teaching exercises. This work included an experimental film about clocks, which served as an engaging visual introduction to a Grand Rounds presentation on the clock-drawing test, as well as a taped interview with a patient, whose story residents were tasked with piecing together (Silver, 2016). Another correspondent described the use of films like *Still Life: The Humanity of Anatomy* (2001) to prompt first-year medical students to confront and reflect on the process of working with human cadavers.[30] An elective course for fourth-year medical students on film and mental illness addressed both questions of accuracy and larger philosophical questions such as "How have such cinematic representations shaped our personal responses, cultural beliefs, and social policies regarding the mentally ill and those who care for them? And can film be used to advocate for mentally ill persons without exploiting them?"[31,32] Taken together, these isolated initiatives begin to trace the contours of an alternative approach to film-based learning, one that takes as its focus the implications—personal, societal, and cultural—of looking at another. They suggest the medium's capacity to gesture toward ineffable, subjective experiences and to create a space for the safe confrontation of difficult material. We discuss these qualities in greater detail next.

Properties and Applications of Film: The Gaze

Film theorist and cultural critic Siegfried Kracauer, writing in the wake of World War II and its attendant atrocities, likened the film screen to "Athena's polished shield," used to reflect that which would be too horrifying to confront directly.[33] In Greek mythology, Athena's shield, gifted to Perseus, enabled him to indirectly view and thus behead the Gorgon Medusa, whose face was said to turn those who gazed upon it to stone. Cinema fulfills a similar function by presenting to spectators mediated images of reality, including taboo material like death and dying, as suggested by the previous cadaver example. In bearing witness to these "reflections of horror," Kracauer argues, "we redeem horror from its invisibility behind the veils of panic and imagination."[33] The documentary *Dying at Grace* (2003), for example, which follows in unflinching close-up the final moments of five individuals with terminal cancer, allows those planning to work in a hospice setting to familiarize themselves with the materiality—the look, feel, and sound—of the process of dying. While postgraduate students are not immune from the daily direct confrontation of "dreadful" phenomena, film offers a safe and low-stakes space to debrief and process these encounters. Death, defined as the absence of being and meaning, tests the limitations of film as a representational medium. It also calls attention to certain ethical issues related to the act of looking at another person, as the act of looking at a person become a body constitutes objectification. A closer examination of films about death and dying will help elucidate important properties of the medium and its relevance to medical education.

The concept of "the gaze" is central to both theories of film and medical knowledge. In *The Birth of the Clinic*, Michel Foucault defines the "clinical gaze" as one that necessarily considers the patient "in parenthesis" relative to disease in service of objectivity and "truth."[34] "Truth" in this context reflects ideas and ideals informed by social and cultural hierarchies.[2] The act of seeing is thus implicated in power inequities between physician (seer) and patient (seen). Film theorist Laura Mulvey similarly traces a connection between systems of power and structures of looking. In her seminal essay "Visual Pleasure and Narrative Cinema," Mulvey adopts a psychoanalytic framework to argue that patriarchal ideology has shaped the formal system of classical Hollywood cinema.[35] This model presumes a heterosexual male spectator who derives pleasure from (a) gazing at a passive female who connotes "to-be-looked-at-ness" and (b) identifying with an active male character, the "bearer of the look." Identification is facilitated both visually (e.g., through point-of-view shots that align viewers with the perceptual perspective of a male protagonist) and narratively (e.g., through the agency of a goal-driven male protagonist whose actions drive the plot). For both Foucault and Mulvey, the act of seeing is empowering, pleasurable, and associated with a sense of mastery; it reaffirms one's sense of self as well as the dominant ideology. Cinema is of value to medical educators for the opportunity it provides to interrogate the clinical gaze and to seek a radical alternative: a gaze characterized by ambiguity, shared humanity, selflessness, and identification with powerlessness. Both are required to promote the humanistic capacities of critical reflection and empathy.

In addition to foregrounding matters of the mind, much of the literature cited here tends to emphasize films that are commercial, North American, narrative, and feature-length to the relative exclusion of the wealth of film media that fall outside of these parameters, including short-form content, documentaries that seek to amplify the patient voice, consumer-created videos distributed online through video-sharing platforms like YouTube, and non-narrative, experimental cinema. The latter—which can challenge assumptions about meaning, closure, and representation—is "useful" precisely because it is "useless" and allows students to wrestle with and incorporate the experience of uncertainty. In an essay titled "Experimental Film as Useless Cinema," film scholar Mike Zryd describes the productive frustration that can result from encountering experimental cinema in the classroom.[36] While such films might be met with resistance from students and residents in comparison to engaging narrative film—for failing to meet standards of pleasure or clarity, for example—the processing of this resistance through discussion, Zryd argues, forces students to consider their activities as spectators as well as the unconscious biases and expectations that underpin them. For residents, this act of consideration should also extend to clinical encounters. Therefore, experimental cinema can "become useful by being anti-useful, by opposing utilitarian, instrumental pedagogy in favor of an approach that invites open, complex, and sometimes discomfiting experience." This approach requires a certain investment, from both educators and students, in a radical conception of learning and its objectives. The classroom shifts "from a place where knowledge is theoretically hypodermically inserted to one where the very forms and limits of knowledge are ideally debated and contested." Thus, enhanced critical thinking can be one of the learner benefits of such approaches. For these reasons, "experimental" films, or simply films that defy and point up conventions of mainstream narrative cinema (e.g., closure, linearity, meaning), provide a good case study for illustrating the value of the medium in the context of postgraduate medical education.

Building upon this theoretical foundation, we will now further outline a model of film-based learning that pays equal due to both content and form by way of a few representative examples.

Beyond Illustration: A Collaborative Approach to Film-Based Learning

The Cinema Medica film series, offered now over for five years through the University of Toronto Health, Arts and Humanities program, explores topics related to healthcare through the curated selection and facilitated discussion of films ranging from Hollywood blockbusters to the independent avant-garde to micro-budget student productions. The film texts vary per the specific needs and interests of the audience as well as the educational objectives determined by the organizers and any formalized partnerships, though the presentation format and discussion framework remain constant. All sessions are co-led by a representative from both the humanities (cinema studies) and medicine (psychiatry), modeling an interdisciplinary perspective that asks all participants to exceed their specialized frames of reference. Guest speakers such as filmmakers, "subject experts," and persons with lived experience are occasionally invited to participate in the experience, and their contributions are held in dialogue with other components of the event. One session titled "Perspectives on Mental Health" featured a selection of student short films about mental health solicited from local undergraduate film production programs.

Taken together, the films represented a diversity of experiences, topics, and formal strategies rather than a single, coherent portrait of mental health and illness. The student-filmmakers were present to provide context for and participate in a discussion about their work, but they were also able to ask their audience of healthcare students questions in return. Other sessions have addressed skills, attitudes, and values related to interprofessional collaboration, with allied health students viewing a film and then breaking into small, diverse groups to discuss emerging themes in conversation with their own experiences; the intersection between medical ethics and the ethics of documentary intervention, particularly as this pertains to marginalized and vulnerable groups; and film as a tool of advocacy for policy change and stigma reduction.

Close Reading: Irrational, Material Illness in *Son frère* (2003)

Patrice Chéreau's *Son frère* (2003) foregrounds the act of looking at illness, and as such it can be used to point up and subvert the "clinical gaze." On the narrative level, it presents a counterpoint to classical depictions of death and dying, which is coded as meaningful and follows a predictable course. Graeme Harper and Andrew Moor chart this course, drawing a correspondence between the popular expectation that illness is teleological and the classical narrative arc: "An equilibrium of good health is disrupted; incapacities caused by the illness's symptoms present themselves as obstacles; closure is achieved when the symptoms are eradicated or, if the illness proves fatal, the narrative may engineer a 'good death,' a noble end with consequence."[2] Conversely, the plot of *Son frère* is organized around the unpredictable ebb and flow of the main character, Thomas's, gradual deterioration from an nonspecific platelet disorder, as witnessed by his estranged brother Luc. It does not offer a linear sequence, beginning near the end of Thomas's life and presenting the events before and after his surgery in nonchronological order. His condition improves and worsens repeatedly. Whereas many narrative films, particularly Hollywood films, tend to reduce death to a plot device or a means of closure, this is a film about the duration and physicality of the dying process. It develops slowly through a series of long takes (i.e., unedited shots of an extended duration) in which very little happens or is said.

It abandons illusions of medical mastery and casts a critical eye toward the objectification that characterizes the "clinical gaze." Providing a counterpoint to illness tropes in Western media that seek to ennoble the patient-character in the face of suffering by framing stoicism as a virtue, an irate Thomas complains to the medical staff: "You poke and prod me all over. But you don't seem to be getting anywhere. Is it too much to ask, to feel like more than a hunk of meat?" His complaint is that his illness does not have a scenario. The doctors can only confirm what it is not: leukemia, AIDS, and so on. They keep trying different treatments to no avail. Medical intervention never develops a real narrative. After an unsuccessful splenectomy, Thomas's doctor informs him that his body continues to destroy his platelets "for reasons [they] don't understand" and that he could die of a sudden hemorrhage at any time, or perhaps not at all. Chance and contingency supersede the classical conventions of predictability and destiny.

This narrative is supported by a formal emphasis on the body in decline, which compensates for and highlights the failure of language and reason in such circumstances. It negotiates between the elusive and the concrete. The camera, usually tethered to Luc's perspective, lingers on bruised and decaying flesh, blood, and hair in the close-up. It fixes on Thomas's lesioned foot; a syringe that pierces his flesh, drawing several vials of blood; and his torso being shaved in preparation for an operation in a passage lasting over six minutes. After the operation, the camera slowly scans his scarred body, tracing a catheter to a bag collecting urine beneath his bed. This is neither a clinical nor voyeuristic gaze but a gaze that empathetically bears witness to a shared experience of suffering and mortality. Thomas asks Luc to "pay attention to everything."

Luc silently observes his brother's medical procedures and physical transformation throughout, saying very little. His mother also struggles to find meaningful words in the face of Thomas's illness. She chatters idly during an early scene in which the family gathers at his bedside, describing her commute in detail while a subjective camera (i.e., point-of-view shot) registers Thomas's disinterest. Straying from his mother's image, the camera (Thomas's gaze) moves in on the breathing, bruised body of a fellow patient being examined in the adjacent bed. This material event ruptures the narrative, and the image track takes precedence over dialogue in this moment. *Son frère* allows residents to contemplate death as an often senseless and material reality rather than rationalizing it away by imbuing it with meaning or moral purpose. This may more closely reflect residents' clinical experiences with death than traditional portrayals of terminal illness in mainstream cinema.

Images of Luc turning or pausing to inspect some material detail are intercut throughout to underline his perceptual activity. Our screen surrogate, he embodies a gaze that is uncomfortable and powerless, implicating him in the illness of another. The destabilizing potential of this confrontation—our confrontation—becomes apparent in a hallucination scene. After Luc's partner advises him to contemplate his relationship with Thomas because they "are sharing something important," Luc enters Thomas's surgical recovery room and asks simply to watch. The camera moves from a close-up of Thomas's face, covered in tubes and electrodes, to one of Luc, staring at his brother's unconscious form. It then enters his mind, cutting to a point-of-view shot of Luc wandering through a house. He sees himself in Thomas's place, on life support. The film cuts between Luc gazing at his ill counterpart and Luc on the bed. He sees the unseeable through Thomas: his own death. Returning to Thomas's room, the scene concludes with an extreme close-up of Luc's eyes, explicitly linking vision in the process of identifying with a dying subject. As terminal illness makes visible the subject's contingent relation to the body, it also renders malleable the distinction between subject and object, self and other.

Overall, *Son frère* demonstrates how narrative and form work together to engage viewers in a cinematic experience. Duration, nonlinear narrative, and camera techniques (i.e., structures of looking) come together in a system that confronts certain objectifying tendencies in both medicine and cinema to repurpose these to articulate the limits of knowledge and mastery. In watching and debriefing a film like *Son frère*, students can cultivate a comfort in not-knowing and disorder.

Practical Considerations

Screenings can take many forms. Either an entire film or excerpts from films are shown depending on learning objectives, participant availability, and educator resources available (see sample lesson plans referenced in the website, http://cahh.ca/resources/ouplesson-plans/). Following a screening, the organizers facilitate a discussion amongst the audience members, which can take the form of preprepared specific questions, more open-ended prompts, or an open call for observations. Facilitation style should reflect the number of attendees. In smaller groups of 20 or fewer trainees, the discussion can occur within the whole group. For larger groups, it can be helpful to break into small groups of 3 to 10. This works best when there are facilitators present to guide each small group, though prepared handouts of discussion prompts can suffice. After a designated amount of time, the larger group can reconvene to share overall thoughts and outcomes.

Public film screenings require the presenter to obtain screening rights for film material, even within the context of non-profit educational events. For educators working in institutional settings, university libraries often have media holdings and obtain licenses permitting the use of materials for on-campus educational purposes.

If educators choose to screen a film not included in this catalogue, they are obligated to obtain screening rights. Medical librarians at the hospital or medical school can often assist in this process, helping to secure screening rights for non-profit teaching purposes. This can also be accomplished independently by contacting the film's distributor, if applicable, and negotiating a screening fee. Many independent or student films are not represented by distribution companies. In this case, filmmakers may be contacted directly to secure screening rights and presentation materials, often free of charge or for a nominal fee. Video-sharing websites like YouTube and Vimeo can be a great resource for identifying accessible, consumer-created content (e.g., video diaries documenting treatment and recovery, spoken word performances related to illness experiences). In addition to being cost effective, seeking out such titles allows educators to broaden the scope of content under consideration, amplifying alternative perspectives and discourses.

In selecting a venue, audiovisual requirements and seating are important. Most universities will have auditoriums or dedicated screening rooms, although these may be on campus and distant from teaching hospitals, which can adversely affect attendance. Hospitals sometimes have rooms equipped with projectors, speakers, and Blu-ray/DVD players, but their setup may make it difficult for all attendees to have a clear view of the screen. Some educators also host informal movie clubs out of their homes. Whenever possible, stagger seating and project content above the eyeline, particularly if subtitles are used. It is important to test equipment beforehand, as technical issues can easily undermine an otherwise well-planned event. Another important concern is accessibility. In selecting a venue, ascertain how accessible it is for those with limited mobility. Consider the possibilities of supplementing content with descriptive audio, captions, and sign language interpretation. If films contain emotionally charged or potentially triggering content, it is recommended that this be flagged for participants both in promotional announcements and at the start of a session.

Finally, partnering with community organizations and university groups and departments outside of healthcare (e.g., film studies, film production) can increase attendance, optimize available resources, and contribute to the diversity and quality of programming. In the past, we have collaborated with the Toronto International Film Festival and Dignitas International on joint events. Through partnership with the former, we have also organized a reflective filmmaking workshop wherein psychiatry residents created a short documentary on the topic of resilience in residency. This session was led by a professional filmmaker who edited the collective piece, and participants were involved in every stage of the creative process. The process was as important, if not more important, than the final product. Residents took turns being in front of and behind the camera, interviewing one another and being interviewed. Throughout, they were asked to reflect on their relative feelings of control and vulnerability, drawing connections between their roles and experiences on the documentary and those in the clinical interview setting. It is beyond the purview of this chapter to provide a fuller examination of film-making and its potential applications to medical education, but it warrants mentioning as another method for incorporating the medium.

Conclusion

This chapter reviewed previous work pertaining to the use of cinema in medical education, highlighting the relative dearth of studies focusing on postgraduate education. We then advocated for a novel theoretical orientation, wherein film can encourage learners to confront the "clinical gaze" that permeates both film and medicine, instead working through the role of not-knowing in medicine. *Son frère*, a film dealing with chronic illness and death, was profiled. Its nonlinear narrative construction and subjective cinematography, used to convey its characters' powerlessness as an unidentified disease progresses unpredictably, encourage learners to face head-on the limits of medical knowledge. Film is an immersive medium, making it particularly suited to cultivating learners' familiarity with a position of not-knowing. Postgraduate medical trainees, who have accumulated significant clinical experience and are developing their identities as practitioners, are best poised to explore this through film viewing and discussion.

A sample curriculum to accompany this chapter can be found online at http://cahh.ca/resources/ouplesson-plans/.

References

1. Wedding D, Boyd M, Mary A, Niemiec RM. *Movies and Mental Illness: Using Films to Understand Psychopathology*. Boston: Hogrefe & Huber; 2005.
2. Harper G, Moor A. *Signs of Life: Cinema and Medicine*. New York: Wallflower Press; 2005.
3. Colt HG, Quadrelli S, Friedman LD. *The Picture of Health: Medical Ethics and the Movies*. London: Oxford University Press; 2011.
4. Alexander M, Lenahan P, Pavlov A. *Cinemeducation: Using Film and Other Visual Media in Graduate and Medical Education—Volume 2*. London: Radcliffe; 2012.
5. Darbyshire D, Baker P. A systematic review and thematic analysis of cinema in medical education. *Med Humanit*. 2012;(38):28–33. doi:10.1136/medhum-2011-010026
6. Law M, Kwong W, Friesen F, Veinot P, Ng SL. The current landscape of television and movies in medical education. *Perspect Med Educ*. 2015;4(5):218–224. doi:10.1007/s40037-015-0205-9
7. Carroll N. Film/mind analogies: The case of Hugo Munsterberg. *J Aesthet Art Crit*. 1996;46(4):293–304.
8. Fritz GK, Poe RO. The role of a cinema seminar in psychiatric education. *Am J Psychiatry*. 1979;136(2):207–210. doi:10.1176/ajp.136.2.207
9. Hyler SE, Schanzer B. Using commercially available films to teach about borderline personality disorder. *Bull Menninger Clin*. 1997;61(4):458–468.
10. Rosenstock J. Beyond *A Beautiful Mind*: Film choices for teaching schizophrenia. *Acad Psychiatry*. 2003;27(2):117–122. doi:10.1176/appi.ap.27.2.117
11. Bhugra D. Teaching psychiatry through cinema. *Psychiatrist*. 2003;27(11):429–430.

12. Kalra G. Teaching diagnostic approach to a patient through cinema. *Epilepsy Behav.* 2011;22(3):571–573. doi:10.1016/j.yebeh.2011.07.018

13. Tarsitani L, Brugnoli R, Pancheri P. Cinematic clinical psychiatric cases in graduate medical education. *Med Educ.* 2004; 38(11):1181. doi:10.1111/j.1365-2929.2004.01993.x

14. Hyler SE, Remien R. Using commercial films to teach about AIDS. *J Pract Psychiatry Behav Heal.* 1998;4(4):230–235.

15. Farré M, Bosch F, Roset PN, Baños J-E. Putting clinical pharmacology in context: The use of popular movies. *J Clin Pharmacol.* 2004;44(1):30–36. doi:10.1177/0091270003260679

16. Welsh CJ. OD's and DT's: Using movies to teach intoxication and withdrawal syndromes to medical students. *Acad Psychiatry.* 2003;27(3):182–186. doi:10.1176/appi.ap.27.3.182

17. Pais de Lacerda A. Medical education: Addiction and the cinema (drugs and gambling as a search for happiness). *J Med Movies.* 2005;1:95–102.

18. Fresnadillo Martínez JM, Amado CD, García Sánchez E, Sánchez García JE. Teaching methodology for the utilization of cinema in the teaching of medical microbiology and infectious diseases. *J Med Movies.* 2005;1(1):17–23.

19. Alexander M, Hall MN, Pettice YJ. Cinemeducation: An innovative approach to teaching psychosocial medical care. *Fam Med.* 1994;26(7):430–433. http://www.ncbi.nlm.nih.gov/pubmed/7926359

20. Wadhwa R, Thakur JD, Cardenas R, Wright J, Nanda A. Synoptic philosophy in a neurosurgical residency: A book and cinema club. *World Neurosurg.* 2013;80(5). doi:10.1016/j.wneu.2012.10.069

21. L. Kaye D, Ets-Hokin E. *The Breakfast Club*: Utilizing popular film to teach adolescent development. *Acad Psychiatry.* 2000;24(2):110–116. doi:10.1176/appi.ap.24.2.110

22. Shapiro J, Elder NC, Schwarzer A. Using the cinema to understand the family of the alcoholic. *Fam Med.* 2002;34(6):426–427.

23. McNeilly DP, Wengel SP. The "ER" seminar: Teaching psychotherapeutic techniques to medical students. *Acad Psychiatry.* 2001;25(4):193–200. http://www.ncbi.nlm.nih.gov/pubmed/11744535

24. Furst BA. Bowlby goes to the movies: Film as a teaching tool for issues of bereavement, mourning, and grief in medical education. *Acad Psychiatry.* 2007;31(5):407–410. doi:10.1176/appi.ap.31.5.407

25. Alexander M. The doctor: A seminal video for cinemeducation. *Fam Med.* 2002;34(2):92–94.

26. Kalra G. Talking about stigma towards mental health professionals with psychiatry trainees: A movie club approach. *Asian J Psychiatr.* 2012;5:266–268. doi:10.1016/j.ajp.2012.06.005

27. Bhugra D. Using film and literature for cultural competence training. *Psychiatr Bull.* 2003;27(11):427–428.

28. Klemenc-Ketis Z, Kersnik J. Using movies to teach professionalism to medical students. *BMC Med Educ.* 2011;11(1):60. doi:10.1186/1472-6920-11-60

29. Lumlertgul N, Kijpaisalratana N, Pityaratstian N, Wangsaturaka D. Cinemeducation: A pilot student project using movies to help students learn medical professionalism. *Med Teach.* 2009;31(7):e327–e332. http://www.ncbi.nlm.nih.gov/pubmed/19811142

30. Kayhan Parsi, JD, PhD, email communication, November 24, 2016.

31. Jones, Tess, MEDS 8040: "Film and Mental Illness," 2016.

32. Tess Jones, PhD, email communication, November 25, 2016.

33. Kracauer S. *Theory of Film: The Redemption of Physical Reality.* Princeton: Princeton University Press; 1997.

34. Foucault M. *The Birth of the Clinic: An Archaeology of Medical Perception.* New York: Routledge; 1963. doi:10.1016/0037-7856(76)90065-2

35. Mulvey L. Visual pleasure and narrative cinema. *Screen.* 1975; 16(3):6–18.

36. Zryd M. Experimental cinema as useless cinema. In: Acland CR, Wasson H, eds. *Useful Cinema.* 1st ed. Durham, NC: Duke University Press; 2011:315–336.

3

Narrative Medicine in Postgraduate Medical Education

Practices, Principles, Paradoxes

SHANNON ARNTFIELD AND KATHRYN HYNES

Introduction

Narrative medicine (NM), as defined by Dr. Rita Charon in her seminal article from 2001, is "medicine practiced with narrative competence [which is] the ability to acknowledge, absorb, interpret and act on the stories and plights of others."[1] Proposed as a "model for empathy, reflection, profession and trust," NM saw rapid uptake across North America through a confluence of four forces. Ideologically, NM was received by scholars as a response to the longstanding call for improving and increasing "humanism" in medicine.[2-5] Strategically, NM was capitalized on by medical educators looking for a means by which to satisfy accreditation standards for skills difficult to teach, such as communication, collaboration, and professionalism.[6-9] Societally, NM resonated with the public in an era that both prioritized the singular experience and enabled increased readership of personal illness narratives through social media. Practically, the establishment of recognized training programs for NM, especially Columbia University's master's program and Boston's Center for Narrative Practice, created increasing numbers of "change agents" who can disseminate knowledge and skill in broad reaching institutions.

I[a] (Shannon Arntfield) am a product of these four forces. Attending medical school at the advent of the CanMEDS revolution, my training was shaped by repeated and explicit messages that we must be more than "medical experts" to take care of patients well. The message was intuitive to me, having been named a "renaissance woman" by pre-med educators who recognized and encouraged my commitment to the arts while I pursued the sciences. My love of literature, writing, and theater had created a deep respect for, and curiosity about, the lived experience. When I started residency and became a witness to human suffering in real time, however, I was deeply disappointed to learn that medical practitioners are not well equipped to come alongside patients during illness or navigate the personal consequences of caring for others. This problem arose, at least in part, from the failure of medical education to explicitly train learners in the skills and knowledge required to engage in the *experience* of illness. This realization led me to pursue the master's of science degree in narrative medicine at Columbia University, which provided a formal platform with which I could teach and study the intersection of narrative and medicine. With funding acquired through the Arnold P. Gold Foundation and an AMS Phoenix Fellowship (see chapter 11 for more information on these funding bodies), I was later able to develop a NM initiative at my institution, one component of which was the development of a mandatory longitudinal curriculum in NM for postgraduate trainees in the ob/gyn department. I have been running the NM curriculum for residents since 2013, and my personal observations of the outcomes for residents includes increased sensitivity to the patient perspective, increased sensitivity and curiosity about the experience of illness, increased recognition of the emotions that influence care relationships and how they manifest (fear, shame,

---

a. The use of the first person throughout the chapter refers to the primary author, Dr. Shannon Arntfield.

loss, guilt, etc.), increased recognition of power dynamics in care and how to navigate them, improved collegiality among residents, increased willingness to acknowledge the cost of caring for others, increased frequency of engaging in self-care, and more frequent and automatic self-reflection. This chapter intends to illuminate how and why NM training can enable these and other outcomes.

The recent path of medical education and my own personal journey led to an invitation to contribute to this book, and what I present here is a practically minded conceptualization of the field of NM *as it relates to educators* in postgraduate medicine. Written with both the novice and the experienced practitioner in mind, I make explicit the *practices* of NM, articulate the tacit *principles* that underpin the work, and identify and explore the *paradoxes* that arise when using this discipline within medical culture. The final portion of the chapter is devoted to resources, teaching suggestions, and sample material that can be used in NM sessions with residents.

The construction of this chapter has drawn on three main sources of material: my own personal experience working with residents as clinician-educator, the peer-reviewed literature, and personal conversations with over 32 North American colleagues currently using NM for resident training. Conversations were necessary because much of the practical residency-based knowledge has not yet appeared in the published literature. What is formally known is that NM has been implemented in postgraduate education (PGE) across the United States and Canada throughout a vast range of programs including family medicine,[10-12] internal medicine,[13-16] surgery,[17,18] oncology,[19] pediatrics,[8] emergency medicine,[20,21] psychiatry,[22,23] obstetrics,[24,25] and neurology.[26] Research conducted within these initiatives has explored narrative medicine as a method for improving communication, reflection, empathy, and development of professional identity, and relevant findings can be found threaded throughout the remainder of this chapter. Narrative approaches have also been studied in the United Kingdom, beginning with the work of Greenhalgh and Hurwitz who suggested "narrative-based medicine" as a framework for approaching patients holistically. Notably, the movement came 10 years prior to the advent of NM in the United States. Greenhalgh and colleagues moved narrative-based medicine forward in a number of ways, including as a method to teach history-taking and interpretation of stories for trainees,[27-30] as a tool to cope with complex unfamiliar contexts, and as a process-based approach to training in capability rather than prescriptive content.[31]

To date, we are not aware of any studies speaking specifically to differences in NM teaching between PGE and undergraduate medical education (UME). Foundational concepts and methods in NM may be universally applied to medical education (UME, PGE), and academic papers do not often make the distinction between implementation at these different stages.[5,32-35] Additionally, there remains a much larger body of literature studying implementation of NM programs in UME, and there are far fewer papers dedicated to PGE research. This may be a reflection of the fact that NM is still not being done as commonly in PGE. The many hurdles of implementation into PGE such as limited didactic time, competing alternatives, and scheduling constraints all contribute to the decreased uptake.[36] Despite this, the transition to residency represents a critical period of change from students into professional work experience. Therefore, efforts to encourage NM programs are highly valuable at this stage to support this progression into the profession.[36,37]

The Intersection between Narrative Medicine and Medical Education

Although this chapter focuses on the *how* of NM, we must spend some time ensuring clarity about *what* is being done and *why*, for the simple reason that advocating for NM requires articulating what it is and why it is needed. It has taken me a long time to do this succinctly in my own institution. I offer here that which has been most useful to me when approaching my colleagues and those in leadership. For an exhaustive review of the theory and practices of NM, please refer to Rita Charon's seminal books.[38,39]

The relevance of NM to medical practice and education arises from the *need for story* when providing and receiving care. Healthcare's need for story is most easily understood through the distinction between illness and disease. *Illness* refers to how the sick person and members of the family perceive, live with, and respond to symptoms and disability.[40] Illness is communicated through story. The person who tells the story is the primary expert and the best person to help others understand his or her experience and its significance. *Disease*, in contrast, is the problem from the practitioners' perspective, made through a reconfiguration of the patient's and family's illness experience into narrow problems of altered biological structure or function. Disease is communicated through signs and symptoms. The person who recognizes those signs and symptoms is the primary expert and the best person to help others understand the problem and its significance. When illness is reduced to disease, conflict between the sick person and the care provider may occur because (a) something essential to the story may be lost, (b) experience is not legitimized, (c) key issues may not receive intervention, and (d) expertise regarding the nature of the problem and potential strategies for care may not be shared.[41] Accordingly, learning how to *think with, and listen for, story* is of critical importance for helping healthcare providers establish therapeutic relationships and provide patient-centered care. Story takes on additional importance when understood as a mechanism for sick people to make sense of what is happening to them, navigate their illness, reclaim their voice, and re-engage with others. Story can also assist care providers, who need strategies to address the influence that training and practice has on them as individuals and make meaning from their experiences. The scope of this chapter prevents a broader exploration of these concepts, but they represent foundational knowledge for every practitioner of NM and are critically reviewed by Arthur Frank in his book *The Wounded Storyteller*[41] and Arthur Kleinman's *Illness Narratives*.[40]

Proponents of NM propose that (a) in order to skillfully engage in story, narrative competence is required, and (b) narrative competence can be developed through NM training. Narrative competence is defined as "the capacity to recognize, absorb, interpret, and be moved by stories of illness."[38] It is necessary for care because if practitioners are not moved by someone else's experience, they cannot care for them effectively. The argument receives support from numerous scholars of illness narratives, including Kleinman[40] and Frank,[41] who suggest that care is best when it arises from a dialectic in which the practitioner has "joined with" the patient through the act of listening and then acts *for* them as an ethical response to what has been heard. Narrative competence is critical within this framework because unless one has undergone a personal illness experience, or cared deeply for someone who has, it is difficult if not impossible to appreciate what a person goes through when he or she is sick.

Narrative competence can be developed through training with narrative. By exposing people, through story, to what they themselves have not encountered, learners develop skill in imagining the "interior" experience of others. The theoretical premise underpinning this argument is that reading builds an awareness of intersubjectivity.[38] This theory has recently received support in a *Science* paper[42] in which participants were randomized to reading literary fiction, popular fiction, or nonfiction, and researchers found that participants who read literary fiction achieved higher scores on tests measuring empathy, social perception, and emotional intelligence. Scores were not elevated in the other groups, and authors hypothesized that reading literary fiction forces readers to make inferences about characters and be sensitive to emotional nuance and complexity because the genre leaves more to the imagination, unsettles the expectations of the reader, and "challenges their thinking."

I have put these concepts together in Figure 3.1 which illustrates how NM works. The dependent relationships among the underpinning premises highlights how the entire argument for NM falls apart if the foundational statement that *story is important* is not accepted. Importantly, the current system of medical education is set up to be in conflict with this foundational statement by training learners to think in terms of disease rather than illness. I believe

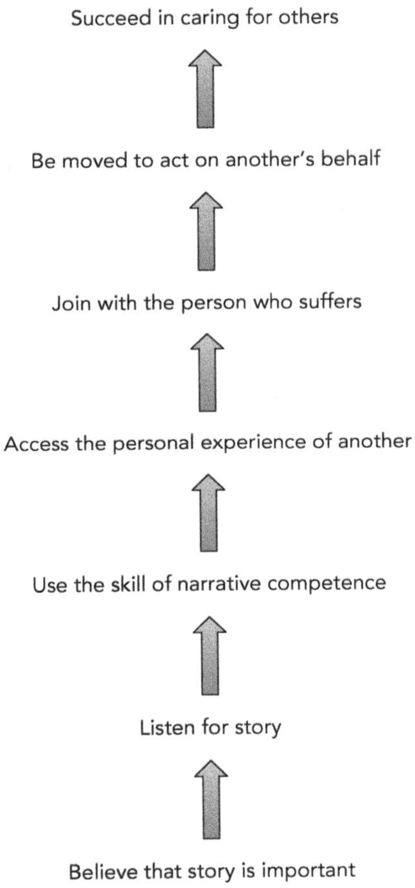

Succeed in caring for others

Be moved to act on another's behalf

Join with the person who suffers

Access the personal experience of another

Use the skill of narrative competence

Listen for story

Believe that story is important

FIGURE 3.1. How narrative medicine works.

this is the primary reason that NM has not been fully integrated in medical education. Until the system recognizes and promotes *illness* as a fundamental construct for patient care and training, *story*, and therefore NM, can have no central purpose in medical education.

Explaining Narrative Medicine to the "Uninitiated" Medical Colleague

It can be difficult to explain the use of NM for training to medical colleagues, who may have no familiarity with the concept, preconceived notions, or perceptions that the field is too foreign to be relevant or accessible.[9] I have found it effective to offer the educational comparison of simulation. In this comparison, both narrative and simulation advocate for exposure to clinical correlates in advance of, or in addition to, the training residents obtain in "real time" with patients.[43] Both approaches work to reveal and improve upon the existing skill set a resident has to attune to, interpret, and respond to an event or story. Both rely on a narrative framework written by someone else that invites the participant into an experience. Both require the suspension of disbelief for the exercise to be successful. Both require a skilled facilitator. And both require a group setting in which colleagues' function as observers *and* participants, which ensures that multiple viewpoints are available, represented, and voiced.

Practices

NM consists of three primary practices, all of which are communal and typically facilitated: the sharing of a narrative, close reading with discussion, and reflective writing (RW). All practices arise as a response to this central concept: "To know what patients endure at the hands of illness and therefore to be of clinical help requires that doctors *enter* the worlds of their patients, if only imaginatively, and to see and interpret these worlds from the patients' point of view."[38]

The Sharing of a Narrative

Sharing a narrative in a group setting enhances learning because the reader (listener), the writer (speaker), and the text (story itself) all have an opportunity to be seen and heard through multiple viewpoints. When those viewpoints are exchanged, appreciation for and learning about the reader's stance, the writer's stance, and the textual elements of ambiguity, uncertainty, and nuance increases. Additional clinical relevance is achieved by virtue of how the text illuminates and sensitizes the reader to the narrative features of medicine, which are outlined by Charon.[38]

When choosing a narrative to be shared with a group, the most common form is written, whether poetry or prose. Educators working with residents often use multiple alternatives, including graphic novels, comics, spoken-word, oral history, theater, film, music, and various forms of visual art. Given that other chapters of this book address many of these, only written narratives are discussed here.

If the narrative is short (i.e., three pages or less) and the group size relatively small and familiar, the traditional method of sharing the narrative is for the full text to be read aloud by two different readers, ideally one male and one female, as this provides a contrast of voice and delivery. If the text is very long or the group very large or unfamiliar, representative excerpt(s) chosen by the facilitator ahead of time are read aloud by multiple individual participants who read successive segments of the text in turn.

To promote intersubjectivity, the best type of narrative for training sessions are literary—that is, well-crafted narratives that incorporate elements of ambiguity, uncertainty, and critical thinking—because they ensure there is sufficient material for examination, discussion, and learning. When working with residents, most educators favor shorter pieces that do not require prereading; this tends to improve attendance and internal motivation, increase participation, and avoid the discussion breakdown that can occur when some participants do not preread (or read but do not remember) longer narratives. Numerous resources exist for finding and mining narrative material, with some specific examples provided in the appendix.

Close Reading

Close reading is the act of intentionally exploring how a narrative has been constructed and is intended to help a reader understand how a text achieves its meaning. The beauty of the practice of close reading is that it simultaneously illuminates not only the literary elements of a text but also the characteristics of the reader, both of which influence what is ultimately heard by the reader. By learning to pay attention to both the content of the narrative and the process by which it is told, clinicians can gain transferrable skills to better understand both the *meaning* of a patient's illness narrative and the influence of their skill as a listener.[33,44,45]

Charon suggests that close reading be approached like a drill, much the way a clinical chest x-ray is systematically appraised and read.[38] She starts with examining the frame of the text and moves forward to assess the form, time, plot, and desire of the reading, asking questions of readers along the way. One does not need to be a literary scholar to be able to understand and carry out the practice of close reading; however, training is useful and suggested for session leaders (see appendix for resources). A brief description of each textual element follows, with corresponding definitions provided in Table 3.1. The task of the reader, in assessing each literary element, is to examine and appreciate how the various features render the text and enable its meaning.

Examining the *frame* of a text is akin to examining the frame of a photograph: an observer can appreciate the setting, the time frame, the lens that has been used, and the degree of restriction of that lens. Assessing what is visible and how the content has been presented often enables the reader to better appreciate what might be absent from the narrative. The *form* of a text refers to literary and technical features used by the writer to bestow meaning to the text beyond that provided by the words and plot. The genre, visible structure, and diction of the narrative, as well as the stance of the narrator and the writer's use of metaphor and allusion, all contribute to form. Identifying these elements is helpful in understanding *how* a text exerts its' influence on the reader. *Time* refers to the temporal structure of a text and is a particularly helpful skill when engaging with literary and clinical narratives, when time may not flow coherently, or when it may run more quickly or more slowly than expected. *Plot* is typically easy to identify but can often be better understood through the practice of close reading because the textual elements that shape the plot become more apparent.

TABLE 3.1 Close Reading Drill

Element	Description/Definition
Frame	The setting, time frame, and lens that has been used
Form • Genre • Visible Structure • Diction • Metaphor • Allusion	Literary features that bestow meaning to the text beyond words and plot • A class or category, characterized by a particular style, form, content • For example, chapters, verses, stanzas • The style of speaking/writing, made up by phrasing, accent, intonation, etc. • A thing regarded as representative or symbolic of something else • An expression designed to call something to mind without mentioning it explicitly; an indirect or passing reference
Time	Temporal structure of a text
Plot	The storyline; the main events that relate in a pattern or sequence
Desire	Sources of motivation that enable/obstruct the reader/writer from engaging

Desire refers to the sources of motivation that enable or obstruct the reader and writer from engaging in story. Why do we read on? What makes us curious? Why do we think the author wrote the piece in the first place? Exploring the need that has (or has not) been satisfied as a result of writing and reading can help readers critically assess both what they have taken away from a narrative as well as the accuracy of that impression.

For the literary scholar, close reading will be second nature. For medical educators, however, who last discussed the influence of metaphor on a text during their bachelor's degree, the practice can be daunting at first. To assist those of you in the latter group who might appreciate having a practical approach to fall back on when facilitating the practice of close reading with residents, Box 3.1 offers a variety of practical questions that can be used to

BOX 3.1 Practical Guide to Facilitate the Practice of Close Reading*

- What do you think this story about?
  - +/− who is this about?
- Describe the "narrative arc" of this story.
- What sort of mood does this story set/leave you in?
  - Can you identify any of the mechanisms in the text that works to achieve that effect?
- What do you notice about the way this story was written?
  - You can cue participants to look at the visible structure of the piece (i.e., the stanzas of a poem), the diction (which can influence tone), the punctuation and language (which can influence the tone and pace of the reading), the use of metaphor and allusion, the voice of the author, the way the text might play to the senses of smell/taste/touch, etc.
  - Alternatively, ask participants to reread the piece silently, using a pen or pencil, and circle words, underline text, or highlight sections that stand out to them; then discuss these aspects. To build narrative knowledge, guide participants toward recognizing the elements of the close reading "drill" when they come up spontaneously.
- What elements of the text bestow meaning to the narrative, other than plot?
- Does anything seem left out of the text? How does that affect the narrative and your experience of it?
- Is there anything about the text that informs you about
  - The author?
  - The authors stance toward the characters?
  - The setting, time frame, or scope of the narrative?
- Did any aspect of the story, or the writing, surprise you?
- Is there anything about the piece that does not make sense to you, or confuses you?

---

*Ensure you provide time and space with each question to allow a number of different responses to be shared, in order to guarantee that multiple perspectives are presented; this process allows the narrative to be more fully appreciated and understood and simultaneously reveals the biases of one's professional and personal background.

get the conversation started and to encourage shared reflection on the piece. The table was developed through personal experience, NM training, and conversations with colleagues in the field.

Reflective Writing

As a practice of NM, RW is a textually situated act—meaning that it is often grounded by a shared narrative, informed by the process of close reading, guided by a writing prompt, and contextualized by the writers' own stories that rise up and resonate with what has been heard—the act is a landing space for *response*.

In the process of responding, *discovery* is a delightful and common experience that practitioners often find to be one of the most rewarding aspects of NM. Beyond that which has already been discussed and illuminated during reading and discussion, the process of privately putting pen to paper allows for powerful intersections between "self" and "other" to become visible.

Additional discoveries can be made when RW is shared with the group, because the writer (speaker), reader (listener), and text (RW) all have an opportunity to be seen and heard through multiple viewpoints, which increases learning. Extending upon the practice of close reading of the original narrative, listeners can be taught to listen and respond to the reflection in a way that keeps discussion focused on the *text;* this tends to prevent discussion from derailing into intrusive or personal questions directed toward the author and allows the story to remain in the hands of its teller.

RW in NM is typically guided through the use of a writing prompt. Prompts tend to be written "in the shadow" of the text, which means they are constructed with the themes, mood, imagery, or style of the narrative in mind. This supports the writer's reflections to remain grounded in the text and responsive to all that has arisen during subsequent examination and discussion. The appendix at the end of this chapter contains examples of writing prompts that have been created in the shadow of a corresponding narrative for those unfamiliar with this practice. It should be noted that many educators use writing prompts without a corresponding literary piece to good effect, incorporating themes of practice (like CanMEDS roles) or as a part of reflective portfolio entries.

The practice of RW in NM must be distinguished from the various uses of RW in medical education. Much has been written about the utility, limitations, use, and abuse of RW in the latter forum.[10,12,21,24,45–55] In the world of NM, however, the practice of RW should be understood as a specific *method of representing and discovering* all the observations, ideas, questions, and feelings that have been stirred up through the sharing and close reading of a story. As a NM colleague once put it, RW is like a "lightening rod" that allows the energy created through narrative engagement and close reading to be channeled, grounded, and reabsorbed (Caitlyn Chase, MSc, classroom conversation, March 2010).

The practice is not always easy or familiar for residents. The demands of clinical service can limit and frustrate residents' attempts to write or reflect. The constant striving in clinical service can create "performance" habits in residents that inhibit them from entering into a mode of transparency and journeying during RW. The fact that most residents come from a science background means that writing may be an unfamiliar task. Colleagues in the field frequently shared that residents' reluctance to engage in RW initially is one of the larger hurdles when first starting out. However, educators also observed that many residents find the opportunity and dividends of writing to be one of the most satisfying aspects of NM practice, and this draws them back for further experience.

Principles

Underpinning the practices of NM are three major principles: the work should be (a) experiential, (b) relational, and (c) programmatic. When applied, these principles enable and fortify the practices of NM; when undermined, they restrict and threaten the practices of NM. I review each principle in turn, comment on facilitating and obstructing forces, and suggest actions educators can take to cultivate the principles. Table 3.2 provides a summary of this information.

TABLE 3.2 An Overview of the Principles of Narrative Medicine and Their Influences Forces

Principles	Obstructing Forces	Facilitating Forces	How Educators can Cultivate
Experimental	Skepticism Performance anxiety Frequent interruptions (pagers) Insufficient time (less than 60min)	Skilled and credible facilitator Suspension of disbelief Self-discovery ("aha" moment) Relevant/sufficient content for reflection • Literary fiction • Concepts relevant to clinical context	Orienting residents to nature/purpose Establishing a "third space" for session Short readings/no prereadings 60- to 90-min sessions "Five Rules for Writing" Variable methods for reflection
Relational	Culture of clinical distance Culture of power and intimidation Too many participants (>20) Lack of familiarity among participants Infrequent opportunities to engage	Skilled and credible facilitator The power of the work itself Permission to be • Human • Creative • Vulnerable	Recognition/naming of power/authority Lead by example (offer relationality) Use of teaching dyads (humanities-MD) Option to leave if the session is mandatory Emphasize relevance of "illness experience"

(continued)

TABLE 3.2 Continued

Principles	Obstructing Forces	Facilitating Forces	How Educators can Cultivate
Programmatic	Lack of support (faculty/ department)	Culturally supportive institution	Develop a community of practice
	Lack of funding/remuneration	Senior leader who values the work	Embed sessions into formal curriculum
	Lack of access to curricular time	Funding	Obtain evaluations for every session
	Tenuous position for champion	Faculty development	Consider certificates
	Isolated champion	Patience (long view)	Engage in research
	Competing priorities	Enthusiasm	Top-down/bottom-up approach
	No mechanism to distribute across PGE	Resilience	Use curriculum to address local needs
			Apply for internal and external funding

NM Should Be Experiential

Similar to medical training, NM uses an apprenticeship model for teaching where learning occurs through "doing." Educators in both fields understand that practical skills cannot be honed only by studying theory or watching others;[10,16,56] rather, there is a need for a personal, hands-on experience that is relevant, bidirectional, and transferrable.[47,57] In NM, this is achieved through the practice of sharing literary narratives, close reading, and RW, all of which foster dialogic exploration and self-discovery.[58] The most important need that is satisfied through experiential learning is the "aha moment," when participants come to personally know the purpose and benefits of the practice; these opportunities are necessary for building momentum and internal motivation for continued engagement.[50]

A number of factors influence the capacity of NM educators to facilitate experiential learning. Expectations of participants are among the most important. If sessions are optional, these play a relatively minor role because learners, by virtue of self-selecting the opportunity, typically understand the nature and purpose of the session. For mandatory NM sessions, however, there can be a significant discrepancy between the expectations of the learner and the educator, particularly when sessions occur during protected academic time (i.e., academic half-day). In this postgraduate context, residents are most accustomed to didactic teaching focused on the "medical expert" role where learning is unidirectional, hierarchical, and performance-focused. Educators must realize that it is a significant hurdle for trainees to adjust to "process-based" learning that (a) focuses on *how* care is provided, rather than *what* care is provided, and (b) relies on an interactive, noncompetitive environment that is not performance-based.

To be effective in teaching NM, educators must cultivate the principle of experiential learning. An introductory session that reviews the purpose and methods of NM is helpful for orienting residents to the nature of the work. However, this should occur in conjunction with the opportunity to practically engage in narrative and reflection in order to ensure that residents personally experience the benefits of training.[59] I offer residents the opportunity to read and discuss a written narrative of my own journey through residency training, which tends to establish relevance and avoids the introductory session becoming didactic and theoretical. I also find it helpful to compare sessions to simulation training, which creates a frame of reference for the work and normalizes the need for "suspended disbelief" during sessions.[34] Ronna Bloom, who is the Poet in Residence at Mount Sinai Hospital in Toronto, purposefully names the atmosphere for narrative work as a "third space" which is "not a classroom, and not a coffee shop" (Ronna Bloom, MEd, personal communication, September 14, 2016). Kumagai has also described the importance of the "reflective space" and states it "requires three qualities: safety and confidentiality, an intentional designation of a time apart from the distractions of daily life for reflection and dialogue, and an awareness of the transitional nature—the liminality—of a critically important period of professional identity development."[60] Establishing the learning environment in this way creates a productive space and avoids the session degenerating into either didactic teaching or, alternatively, conversations about clinical care. Bloom also encourages residents to use "five rules for writing" which "are an amalgam of Natalie Goldberg's books and Bloom's own writing practice."[61,62] The rules, described with some humor (see Box 3.2) facilitate RW by helping residents step back from the "performance" mentality

---

BOX 3.2 Five Rules for Writing

1. Keep your hand moving.
2. Don't think.
3. Don't censor.
4. You are free to write the worst crap ever.
5. You don't have to share.

that is so pervasive in medical culture and postgraduate training. Another approach to increase engagement during reflection is to offer alternatives to writing, such as graphics and "rich pictures."[63] The rich picture is a form of visual language, which allows for communication through visual elements instead of words. A rich picture can depict both objective and subjective elements of a situation: people, things, ideas, connections, character, feelings, conflicts, and prejudices. Essentially, it is a "*rich* pictorial representation of a situation in all its messiness."[64] For this reason, it is an ideal tool to use when reflecting on complex situations. (See chapter 5 on the use of visual pieces in teaching.)

The setting, duration, and materials provided in NM sessions can also function to facilitate or obstruct experiential learning. Regarding session length, 60 minutes is sufficient but 90 minutes is better. Ideally, sessions occur during "protected time," as it can be extremely challenging for residents to engage imaginatively in narrative, or sustain a mindset of reflection, if they are being constantly interrupted by their pagers or distracted by clinical concern for their patients. Short narratives that can be read collectively by the group within the time frame of the session are preferable to longer narratives that require prereading, for the reasons described earlier. Finally, choosing readings that are relevant to the clinical context of the trainees is helpful, especially in the beginning when engagement can be tentative.[19,24] This does not mean that readings have to contain medical content; rather, they can demonstrate relevance simply by evoking the struggle that residents witness regarding the human condition, either within themselves or their patients. Issues such as hope, resilience, fallibility, futility, suffering, helplessness, fear, shame, loss, grief, and death fulfill this requirement.

NM Should Be Relational

NM asserts that (a) the doctor-patient relationship is at the foundation of care and (b) story is the access point for effectively engaging and enacting that relationship. In keeping with this, NM training uses story to help practitioners develop the necessary skills to *attend to and stay with* the suffering person. Because training occurs through apprenticeship, and uses a bidirectional approach, the process is intrinsically relational.[26,65-67] Illustrating this principle of NM is a quote from a 2013 qualitative study that explored the methods of NM training, where researchers observed that "the process of teaching narrative medicine replicates the very skills it seeks to teach."[9] Specifically, it was felt that "practicing the skills of listening to and valuing both narratives and the people who share them inside the classroom was felt to enable the same process outside the classroom."

A number of factors influence the extent to which an academic environment in PGE can foster the relational principle of NM. Chief among them is the willingness and permission for participants to "be human" and display vulnerability with each other and the session facilitator when engaging in narrative and reflection. This, in turn, is influenced by deep cultural dynamics that arise from at least three different sources: (a) the culture of the hospital or university, (b) the culture of the postgraduate program, and (c) the professional background and relative authority of the facilitator, as well as his or her ability to model appropriate boundaries. If the institution's approach to education and patient care concentrates on disease management at the expense of honoring the illness experience, residents will lack the cues and support to engage relationally. If the culture of the institution or program prioritizes stoicism or clinical distance, then it is harder or takes longer to establish community and trust. Similar challenges exist if the training program operates through power and intimidation. The relative authority of the educator can also influence relationality; this issue is discussed separately in the "credibility paradox" (see later discussion). In my conversations with NM educators in the field, the significance of these factors was discussed repeatedly. It may be useful to select and teach short pieces that explore hierarchy/power as a way of naming some of these dynamics.

The size of the group,[68,69] the familiarity of members of the group with each other, and the extent to which the sessions are embedded into the formal curriculum (specifically whether the time is protected or not and mandatory or not) also influence the relational principle. Ideally, the group is comprised of 8 to 20 participants who meet regularly and develop familiarity with each other. Educators offering elective training sessions found it easier to establish a relational atmosphere than those conducting mandatory sessions. Colleagues working in large programs with many residents struggled more to uphold the relational principle than those working in small programs with fewer residents, both because of logistics (getting participants together) and group dynamics (familiarity among participants).

Educators must be aware of the forces that affect the relational principle, including those arising from the systemic and cultural milieu of their institution and program, as well as hierarchical structures that might exist among residents and between residents and the facilitator. While it may not be possible to eliminate barriers, a relational environment can be cultivated if the relevant issues are named and made visible to all participants. On the other end of the spectrum, it should also be emphasized that this is not a therapy group—there are limits to personal sharing—and that what is told to colleagues cannot be untold.

NM Should Be Programmatic

Many NM educators start out, for various reasons, offering what they can, when they can, to whomever they can. This should not be discouraged because (a) it may be the only way a NM initiative can be launched and (b) individual clinicians and the patients they care for can benefit from the teaching. To broadly influence the process of giving and receiving care across a program or institution, however, NM education should be offered as a mandatory and longitudinal component of training with frequent opportunities for deliberate practice.[20]

It is easier to develop a programmatic approach to training if an educator works within an institution that is culturally supportive of the discipline.[36] Such institutions can be recognized by the presence of: a health humanities department or program, a literature in medicine program, formal "narrative rounds" series, a literary journal, a poet or writer in residence, participation in the practice of parallel charts, creative writing programs, and wellness programs. Educators tend to have access to collaborative relationships, encounter less resistance, and receive more support for their efforts in such institutions. Not surprisingly, this can make the work more effective, sustainable, and enjoyable.

For those of us who start or maintain NM education in institutions that lack an arts-based or "humanities-friendly" context, however, it can be a lonely and vulnerable position to operate from, with potentially less reward and return for one's investment. In such environments, it is important to ensure that NM "change agents" do not remain isolated, because this can lead to discouragement, burnout, and lost opportunities to build capacity. To this end, it is critical for early educators to expend effort identifying and collaborating with local, like-minded individuals. Establishing a community of practice has major dividends, because the group can encourage the change agent, but it can also serve as the first step toward faculty development.[70] Colleagues in the field frequently note these steps are key determinants of sustainability and programmatic change.

To avoid perceptions of irrelevance in the early days of an initiative, it can be helpful to take a "top-down/bottom-up" approach to training, in which practitioners at every stage of education get exposure to NM.[37,71,72] Although this approach requires time and commitment, it sends a clear message that the work is applicable to everyone. Evaluations should be provided at every NM session, because they provide educators with tangible evidence about the value of the teaching and can be used to modify sessions in a way that improves the relational and experiential principles.[12,14,58] In my conversations with colleagues in the field, many emphasized the importance of evaluations and linked them to their ability to acquire protected academic time for NM teaching. If NM teaching can be embedded into the formal curriculum, this lends credibility to the practice and also ensures sufficient frequency and attendance. All of these developments facilitate the programmatic principle. Another approach is for educators to acquire funding for their work, both internal and external (see chapter 11 for funding strategies). Funding serves the practical purposes of remuneration, but it also promotes visibility and legitimacy within an institution. This can help educators garner support from institutional leaders and those in power if it was not available previously. Colleagues in the field were adamant that such support, although not always required in the beginning, was ultimately necessary for long-term success. These and other practical steps for establishing a humanities-based community and program are summarized in chapter 1.

The programmatic principle was felt to be the most influential factor for NM education, according to colleagues in the field.

Paradoxes

Educators are often surprised and can become stymied in their efforts to teach NM by the paradoxes that arise when offering training during PGE. A paradox is "a situation or statement that seems impossible or is difficult to understand because it contains two opposite facts or characteristics."[73] Despite being extremely consequential to an educator's efforts to teach, the paradoxes of NM are, ironically, not immediately obvious. Ideally, educators would be aware of the paradoxes that might affect their work early on and receive help in formulating methods to navigate the issues. Toward that end, I discuss three paradoxes: the implementation paradox, the credibility paradox, and the legitimacy paradox. These are terms of my own conceptualization, formulated through my lived experience as an educator. When reviewing the literature, however, and when speaking with my colleagues in the field, I found ample support for the ideas.

The Implementation Paradox

In this paradox, the practicality of implementing NM methods is in competition with preserving the purity of NM methods. The paradox arises because of pressures of time, logistics, institutional culture, faculty capacity and expertise, and the needs for assessment/ legitimacy. It matters because the paradox cannot be fully resolved and because attempts to navigate it lead to a variety of educational tradeoffs, all of which threaten the integrity of the discipline and/ or its potential for success.

Let me illustrate. This, and later examples, are composites of stories told to me by colleagues in conversation, anonymized and slightly altered to protect identity but reflective of the gist of many anecdotes. Consider an internist who wants to offer NM teaching to residents in his program. He approaches the chair of the department and the program director and receives support for the initiative and protected academic half-day time for teaching. However, there is only one NM-trained faculty member for a department of 60 residents. In an effort to preserve the principles and practices of NM training, he offers faculty development in NM, but pre-existing academic responsibilities are a barrier to colleagues taking on anything extra. The change agent is forced to make one of several educational tradeoffs based on these limitations. First, he can offer elective NM sessions that occur when possible during lunch or non-work hours for interested residents; the trained faculty member can ensure the correct practices are taught and the elective nature of the activity will likely preserve the relational and experiential principles of NM; however, the education will not be programmatic and may lack uptake and legitimacy in the broader PGE context. Second, he could offer mandatory NM sessions that occur only when the trained facilitator can conduct them; this ensures the correct principles are taught; however, the relational and programmatic principles will suffer from the lack of frequency and regularity of sessions, and this will threaten internal motivation among residents, long-term sustainability, and potential for change. Or third, he can modify the methods and goals of the sessions to enable non-NM trained faculty to act as facilitators; this preserves session frequency and regularity but may threaten the integrity of the practices of NM.

A few approaches to this problem have been offered in the literature. Training the trainer is arguably the most important and can be done through workshops, continuing medical education events, or even grand rounds opportunities, all of which can be accredited for further value added. A study examining the impact of a NM workshop on faculty development created an assessment tool consisting of novel trigger video and a narrative skills assessment tool to assess the learning impact of the workshop.[71] The authors found that those who attended the workshop had a more nuanced understanding of narrative than those who did not. Other authors suggest that upper year residents be trained to serve as teaching assistants[74] or that formalized frameworks be used to guide written feedback from mentors.[37] Anecdotally, I am aware that several programs have been successful through their liaisons with humanities scholars, such as those in the departments of English, history, bioethics, and philosophy.

Issues of institutional culture that present limitations to implementation are discussed in the "legitimacy paradox" section.

It is not possible to fully resolve the implementation paradox; rather, educators must attempt to navigate the issue using the resources available to them. General advice is challenging to provide because the paradox is not experienced identically by every practitioner, given that the tension between practicality and purity are by-products of the local context. However, I encourage educators to be intentional about what aspects of the principles and practices of NM they most want to instill and preserve and to be mindful about the consequences of the tradeoffs they are making. This awareness can assist practitioners to decide ahead of time which tradeoffs they are willing to accept and help them anticipate and understand what kinds of difficulties they may subsequently encounter.

The Credibility Paradox

In this paradox, educators whose credibility arises from one professional arena have teaching advantages that are not available to educators whose credibility arises from another professional arena, but both types of credibility are necessary to teach effectively. The paradox arises because educators tend to achieve credibility with residents in one of two ways: from "the inside" through a background in clinical medicine or from "the outside" through a background in the humanities. The paradox matters because educators are simultaneously advantaged and disadvantaged by their professional background in a manner that they cannot resolve and which has implications for their capacity to teach NM effectively.

Educators with a background in the humanities do not tend to have positions of power or authority over residents. This can be advantageous when conducting NM sessions because residents may not feel the same pressure to prove themselves or "perform" for a medically trained educator who, hours before or after a NM session, may be in a supervisory role with the trainee. The permission to appear open and even vulnerable directly promotes the relational and experiential principles of NM, which can enhance learning and internal motivation to continue engaging in sessions. The comparative ease with which a humanities-trained educator can guide NM sessions, based on his or her professional familiarity with literature and the arts, can additionally enhance trainees' development in the practices of NM. Paradoxically, though, educators with a background in the humanities may have *more* difficulty engaging with residents compared to their medically trained counterparts if they are perceived by trainees to have less credibility in the medical realm.[34] If leaders in the department also carry covert/overt bias against humanities trained educators, there can be additional difficulty accessing and sustaining curricular time with trainees. In my conversations with humanities-based scholars working in medical settings, I found that many shared a related struggle of knowing that their position in the hospital or institution was dependent on the changing tides of funding sources and leadership appointments. Several expressed dismay at the shadow this cast for them and others regarding the credibility and sustainability of their work.

For NM educators with a professional background in clinical medicine, there are different types of challenges. Will NM and humanities teaching be taken into account for academic promotions? While actual job security may be less problematic, fluency with the practices of NM may be more difficult depending on the type and duration of NM training obtained. This can pose credibility concerns for both educator and resident and decrease the capacity for trainees to engage experientially with the work. The relative authority of medically trained educators can also pose problems, because the pre-existing hierarchical relationships with residents can compromise the capacity for vulnerability, relationality, and reciprocity during sessions. One particular conversation with a colleague in the field exemplifies some of these issues. She told me that, in her early days of teaching NM as a junior faculty member, she had great sessions with residents who perceived her as a contemporary and engaged in the work, but she struggled to obtain sufficient curricular time based on her position in the department. After obtaining a position of departmental leadership later on in her career, she was able to make the curriculum mandatory, but by that point she had such an authoritative role with residents that she felt unable to run the sessions herself.

The credibility paradox is not resolvable but can be navigated by educators on the basis that NM is inherently interdisciplinary, and, as such, training is best delivered through an interdisciplinary model. Ideally, NM educators are supported and developed through a community of practice and teach as dyads, which is the model used by both faculty and practicum students at Columbia University. In the postgraduate setting where a rich and professionally diverse community may not exist, interdisciplinary teaching can still be achieved practically through the simple pairing of a humanities and a medical scholar. In my conversations with colleagues in the field, many educators described using this approach instinctively, which maximized and supported the expertise and credibility of both teachers and minimized their individual limitations. While such pairings are helpful, they may not always be available because of limitations in remuneration, reciprocity, time, and locations for teaching. The importance of interdisciplinary teaching and training cannot be understated in NM, however, because it is through the illumination of many different lenses that a narrative is fully appreciated and understood. Multiple perspectives cannot be obtained, nor are the biases of one's professional and personal background revealed, when readings are approached through a single dimension.

The Legitimacy Paradox

In this paradox, efforts to achieve one form of legitimacy in NM jeopardize the ability to achieve a second form of legitimacy, and both forms are seen as necessary for success.[49,75] The paradox arises because there are two types of legitimacy that exist for NM in the context of medical education: methodologic legitimacy and assessment legitimacy. In the former, the methods of actually carrying out the principles and practices of NM teaching is what enables the intended outcome, and therefore, methods achieve legitimacy;[44] in the latter, measures of assessment are required to prove that intended outcomes have been achieved, and, as such, measurement achieves legitimacy.[76] The paradox matters because educators can only prioritize one type of legitimacy but are under pressure to achieve both, and the form they choose has major implications to the work.

Outcomes studies of induction of NM programs into PGE have demonstrated the feasibility and importance of NM programs, but causal links between narrative training and key outcomes of interest are still lacking.[77-83] NM has been identified as a tool to promote self awareness,[12,13,46] development of professional identity,[10,36] and communication skills.[20,74] For example, Levine and colleagues[14] completed a one-year study examining personal growth in internal medicine interns after beginning a program of writing narratives monthly. Interns reported deeper reflection and enhanced emotional healing at completion of the study. Winkel and colleagues[24] measured burnout inventory scores for ob/gyn residents before and after introducing a writing workshop into the curriculum. Residents felt the workshops were enjoyable, but trends in burnout scores were not statistically significant. Worley and colleagues[84] who also studied a sample of ob/gyn residents assessed outcomes using professionalism, attitudes, and empathy scales. Results demonstrated nonsignificant improvements in scores after the NM intervention.

Issues affecting outcomes studies to date include being underpowered, relying on small convenience samples of residents to draw conclusions and using loosely structured feedback interviews to discuss the impact of the program. Additional difficulty lies in the methodologic approach to studying outcomes such as empathy, resilience, and personal development. Arguments against the use of reductionist strategies for evaluation have been raised repeatedly, with some scholars arguing that the approach is antithetical to the discipline and others offering insight and suggestions for how to navigate the need for measurement.[75,85–89] The challenges facing outcomes studies in NM research have been summarized in a recent scoping review.[90]

Purists of the field argue that the dividends of NM can only be achieved organically and indirectly—that the so-called "aha moment" arrives only when the participant engages in NM for the purpose of discovery. As such, the only agenda that can be given for a NM session is one of exploration. The NM practitioner knows this from experience. Dictate to participants what they will learn and the session will be dull, disengaging, and static; anticipate that learning can only occur obliquely through engaging with one another and the text, and the process will be dynamic, surprising, and enjoyable. The NM approach to learning is, of course, in direct opposition with the current culture of medical education in which every hour of curricular time has an assigned set of objectives and every form of teaching is matched with a method of assessment.[91] This milieu creates pressure for NM educators to participate in measurement. In some cases, demonstrable outcomes may be required for educators to access or maintain curricular time. If educators cannot or will not engage, this can threaten efforts to make the teaching mandatory, which threatens the work becoming programmatic, which threatens institutional legitimacy, which threatens the capacity to create culture change. On the other hand, agreeing to engage in assessment leaves educators at risk of failing to uphold the principles and practices of NM which begs the question, for whom, and for what reason is the teaching being provided?

Of all the paradoxes of NM, it is legitimacy that has received most attention in the literature and that resonates most deeply with both NM practitioners and naysayers. One example is the effort that has gone into the development and validation of rubrics for assessment of RW[48,92-95] and the corresponding response about the potential for checklists to reduce the complexity and essence of reflection into parts for evaluation.[50,51,96,97] Legitimacy is also the most insidious of the paradoxes because of the tacit manner by which the culture of assessment shapes education. This phenomenon was described in a recent scoping review of research in the medical humanities, which illuminated the manner by which "dominant review methodologies make some functions of medical humanities teaching visible and render others invisible."[90] An important consequence of this phenomenon is that educators may not be conscious that they are choosing a form of legitimacy at all. The paradox of legitimacy has been described by medical humanities scholars as the "danger of instrumentalization," which refers to the overly pragmatic/reductive application of something complex (like a piece of literature or work of art).

The legitimacy paradox cannot be resolved, but educators can make attempts to navigate it in several ways. Accessing curricular time may be easier if educators advocate for the potential for NM to address training needs; these could be needs perceived by the local program or could take the form of pairing sessions with broad accreditation standards such as communication, collaboration and professionalism.[15,17,18,36,74,98-101] In the actual educational session, however, facilitators would be wise to avoid citing these expressed purposes to participants and instead approach the time obliquely using the principles and practices of NM. Similarly, educators should be responsive to requests for objectives but adapt them to honor the process. Understanding the literature surrounding this paradox will enable educators to articulate their concerns clearly to those in leadership and provide a language and external credibility for these concerns. In general, obtaining positive feedback from residents for their experiences in NM sessions may be all that is required to continue providing the teaching. In conversations with colleagues in the field, many report resident feedback to be the most satisfying and achievable form of legitimacy obtainable.

A sample curriculum to accompany this chapter can be found online at http://cahh.ca/resources/ouplesson-plans/.

Acknowledgments

Sincere thanks to Dr. Lorelei Lingard, who graciously helped envision a structure for this chapter and who provided mentorship and feedback on an early draft.

References

1. Charon R. The patient-physician relationship. Narrative medicine: a model for empathy, reflection, profession, and trust. *JAMA*. 2001;286(15):1897–1902.
2. Montgomery K. *Doctors' Stories: The Narrative Structure of Medical Knowledge*. Princeton, NJ: Princeton University Press; 1991.
3. Charon R, Banks JT, Connelly JE, et al. Literature and medicine: contributions to clinical practice. *Ann Intern Med*. 1995;122(8):599–606.
4. Verghese A. The physician as storyteller. *Ann Intern Med*. 2001;135(11):1012–1017.
5. Jones AH. Why teach literature and medicine? Answers from three decades. *J Med Humanit*. 2013;34(4):415–428.

6. Sands SA, Stanley P, Charon R. Pediatric narrative oncology: interprofessional training to promote empathy, build teams, and prevent burnout. *J Support Oncol*. 2008;6(7):307–312.

7. Krasner MS, Epstein RM, Beckman H, et al. Association of an educational program in mindful communication with burnout, empathy, and attitudes among primary care physicians. *JAMA*. 2009;302(12):1284–1293.

8. DasGupta S, Meyer D, Calero-Breckheimer A, Costley AW, Guillen S. Teaching cultural competency through narrative medicine: intersections of classroom and community. *Teach Learn Med*. 2006;18(1):14–17.

9. Arntfield SL, Slesar K, Dickson J, Charon R. Narrative medicine as a means of training medical students toward residency competencies. *Patient Educ Couns*. 2013;91(3):280–286.

10. Clandinin DJ, Cave MT. Creating pedagogical spaces for developing doctor professional identity. *Med Educ*. 2008;42(8):765–770.

11. Shapiro J, Gianakos D. Narrative writing and self-discovery in residency. *Fam Med*. 2009;41(6):395–397.

12. Shaughnessy AF, Duggan AP. Family medicine residents' reactions to introducing a reflective exercise into training. *Educ Health*. 2013;26(3):141.

13. Brady DW, Corbie-Smith G, Branch WT. "What's important to you?": the use of narratives to promote self-reflection and to understand the experiences of medical residents. *Ann Intern Med*. 2002;137(3):220–223.

14. Levine RB, Kern DE, Wright SM. The impact of prompted narrative writing during internship on reflective practice: a qualitative study. *Adv Health Sci Educ*. 2008;13(5):723–733.

15. Ogdie AR, Reilly JB, Pang MWG, et al. Seen through their eyes: residents' reflections on the cognitive and contextual components of diagnostic errors in medicine. *Acad Med*. 2012;87(10):1361.

16. Reisman AB, Hansen H, Rastegar A. The craft of writing: a physician-writer's workshop for resident physicians. *J General Intern Med*. 2006;21(10):1109–1111.

17. Johna S, Woodward B, Patel S. What can we learn from narratives in medical education? *Perm J*. 2014;18(2):92–94.

18. Pearson AS, McTigue MP, Tarpley JL. Narrative medicine in surgical education. *J Surg Educ*. 2008;65(2):99–100.

19. Khorana AA, Shayne M, Korones DN. Can literature enhance oncology training? A pilot humanities curriculum. *J Clin Oncol*. 2010;29(4):468–471.

20. Sklar DP, Doezema D, McLaughlin S, Helitzer D. Teaching communications and professionalism through writing and humanities: reflections of ten years of experience. *Acad Emerg Med.* 2002;9(11):1360–1364.

21. Bernard AW, Gorgas D, Greenberger S, Jacques A, Khandelwal S. The use of reflection in emergency medicine education. *Acad Emerg Med.* 2012;19(8):978–982.

22. Bhuvaneswar C, Stern T, Beresin E. Using the technique of journal writing to learn emergency psychiatry. *Acad Psychiatry.* 2009;33(1):43–46.

23. Deen SR, Mangurian C, Cabaniss DL. Points of contact: using first-person narratives to help foster empathy in psychiatric residents. *Acad Psychiatry.* 2010;34(6):438.

24. Winkel AF, Hermann N, Graham MJ, Ratan RB. No time to think: making room for reflection in obstetrics and gynecology residency. *J Grad Med Educ.* 2010;2(4):610–615.

25. Worly B. Professionalism education of OB/GYN resident physicians: What makes a difference? *Open J Obstet Gynecol.* 2013;3(1):137.

26. Alcauskas M, Charon R. Right brain: Reading, writing, and reflecting: making a case for narrative medicine in neurology. *Neurology.* 2008;70(11):891–894.

27. Greenhalgh T. Narrative based medicine in an evidence based world. *BMJ.* 1999;318(7179):323.

28. Greenhalgh T, Hurwitz B. Why study narrative? *BMJ.* 1999;318(7175):48.

29. Greenhalgh T. Storytelling should be targeted where it is known to have greatest added value. *Med Educ.* 2001;35(9):818–819.

30. Greenhalgh T, Collard A, Begum N. Sharing stories: complex intervention for diabetes education in minority ethnic groups who do not speak English. *BMJ.* 2005;330(7492):628.

31. Fraser SW, Greenhalgh T. Coping with complexity: educating for capability. *BMJ.* 2001;323(7316):799.

32. Aronson L. Twelve tips for teaching reflection at all levels of medical education. *Med Teach.* 2011;33(3):200–205.

33. Blackie M, Wear D. Three things to do with stories: using literature in medical, health professions, and interprofessional education. *Acad Med.* 2015;90(10):1309–1313.

34. Shapiro J, Coulehan J, Wear D, Montello M. Medical humanities and their discontents: definitions, critiques, and implications. *Acad Med.* 2009;84(2):192–198.

35. Kalitzkus V, Matthiessen PF. Narrative-based medicine: potential, pitfalls, and practice. *Perm J.* 2009;13(1):80.

36. Liao JM, Secemsky BJ. The value of narrative medical writing in internal medicine residency. *J Gen Intern Med.* 2015;30(11):1707–1710.

37. Wald HS, Anthony D, Hutchinson TA, Liben S, Smilovitch M, Donato AA. Professional identity formation in medical education for humanistic, resilient physicians: pedagogic strategies for bridging theory to practice. *Acad Med.* 2015;90(6):753–760.

38. Charon R. *Narrative Medicine: Honoring the Stories of Illness.* New York:Oxford University Press; 2008.

39. Charon R, DasGupta S, Hermann N, et al. *The Principles and Practice of Narrative Medicine.* New York:Oxford University Press; 2016.

40. Kleinman A. *The Illness Narratives: Suffering, Healing, and the Human Condition.* New York: Basic Books; 1988.

41. Frank AW. *The Wounded Storyteller: Body, Illness, and Ethics.* Chicago: University of Chicago Press; 2013.

42. Kidd DC, Castano E. Reading literary fiction improves theory of mind. *Science.* 2013;342(6156):377–380.

43. Issenberg SB, McGaghie WC, Petrusa ER, Lee Gordon D, Scalese RJ. Features and uses of high-fidelity medical simulations that lead to effective learning: a BEME systematic review. *Med Teach.* 2005;27(1):10–28.

44. Charon R, Hermann N, Devlin MJ. Close reading and creative writing in clinical education: teaching attention, representation, and affiliation. *Acad Med.* 2016;91(3):345–350.

45. Wear D, Zarconi J, Kumagai A, Cole-Kelly K. Slow medical education. *Acad Med.* 2015;90(3):289–293.

46. Clandinin J, Cave MT, Cave A. Narrative reflective practice in medical education for residents: composing shifting identities. *Medical Educ and Pract.* 2011;2:1–7.

47. Brown JM, McNeill H, Shaw NJ. Triggers for reflection: exploring the act of written reflection and the hidden art of reflective practice in postgraduate medicine. *Reflect Pract.* 2013;14(6):755–765.

48. Aronson L, Niehaus B, Lindow J, Robertson PA, O'Sullivan PS. Development and pilot testing of a reflective learning guide for medical education. *Med Teach.* 2011;33(10):e515–e521.

49. Norrie C, Hammond J, D'Avray L, Collington V, Fook J. Doing it differently? A review of literature on teaching reflective

practice across health and social care professions. *Reflect Pract.* 2012;13(4):565–578.

50. Murdoch-Eaton D, Sandars J. Reflection: moving from a mandatory ritual to meaningful professional development. *Arch Dis Child Educ Pract Ed.* 2014;99(3):279–283.

51. Ng SL, Kinsella EA, Friesen F, Hodges B. Reclaiming a theoretical orientation to reflection in medical education research: a critical narrative review. *Med Educ.* 2015;49(5):461–475.

52. McNeill H, Brown JM, Shaw NJ. First year specialist trainees' engagement with reflective practice in the e-portfolio. *Adv Health Sci Educ Theory Pract.* 2010;15(4):547–558.

53. Toy EC, Harms KP, Morris Jr RK, Simmons JR, Kaplan AL, Ownby AR. The effect of monthly resident reflection on achieving rotation goals. *Teach Learn Med.* 2009;21(1):15–19.

54. Sandars J. The use of reflection in medical education: AMEE Guide No. 44. *Med Teach.* 2009;31(8):685–695.

55. Wear D, Zarconi J, Garden R, Jones T. Reflection in/and writing: pedagogy and practice in medical education. *Acad Med.* 2012;87(5):603–609.

56. Ericsson KA. Deliberate practice and the acquisition and maintenance of expert performance in medicine and related domains. *Acad Med.* 2004;79(10):S70–S81.

57. Devlin MJ, Richards BF, Cunningham H, et al. "Where does the circle end?": Representation as a critical aspect of reflection in teaching social and behavioral sciences in medicine. *Acad Psychiatry.* 2015;39(6):669–677.

58. Kumagai AK. A conceptual framework for the use of illness narratives in medical education. *Acad Med.* 2008;83(7): 653–658.

59. Shapiro J, Lie D. Using literature to help physician-learners understand and manage "difficult" patients. *Acad Med.* 2000; 75(7):765–768.

60. Kumagai AK, Naidu T. Reflection, dialogue, and the possibilities of space. *Acad Med.* 2015;90(3):283–288.

61. Bloom R. The reflecting poem and the use of poetry in health-care education. In: Peterkin A, Brett-MacLean P, eds. *Keeping Reflection Fresh: A Practical Guide for Clinical Educators* Kent, OH: Kent State University Press; 2016:40–43.

62. Goldberg N. *Writing Down the Bones: Freeing the Writer Within.* Boston: Shambhala; 1986.

63. Cristancho S, Bidinosti S, Lingard L, Novick R, Ott M, Forbes T. Seeing in different ways: introducing "rich pictures" in the study of expert judgment. *Qual Health Res*. 2015;25(5):713–725.

64. Armson R. *Growing Wings on the Way: Systems Thinking for Messy Situations*. Axminster: Triarchy Press; 2011.

65. Dickey LA, Truten J, Gross LM, Deitrick LM. Promotion of staff resiliency and interdisciplinary team cohesion through two small-group narrative exchange models designed to facilitate patient- and family-centered care. *J Commun Healthc*. 2011;4(2):126–138.

66. Duggan AP, Vicini A, Allen L, Shaughnessy AF. Learning to see beneath the surface: a qualitative analysis of family medicine residents' reflections about communication. *J Health Commun*. 2015;20(12):1441–1448.

67. Miller E, Balmer D, Hermann MN, Graham MG, Charon R. Sounding narrative medicine: studying students' professional identity development at Columbia University College of Physicians and Surgeons. *Acad Med*. 2014;89(2):335.

68. Coulehan JL, Williams PC. Small-group teaching emphasizing reflection can positively influence medical students' values. *Acad Med*. 2001;76(12):1172–1173.

69. Branch WT, Pels RJ, Harper G, et al. A new educational approach for supporting the professional development of third-year medical students. *J Gen Intern Med*. 1995;10(12):691–694.

70. Branch WT Jr, Frankel R, Gracey CF, et al. A good clinician and a caring person: longitudinal faculty development and the enhancement of the human dimensions of care. *Acad Med*. 2009;84(1):117–125.

71. Liben S, Chin K, Boudreau JD, Boillat M, Steinert Y. Assessing a faculty development workshop in narrative medicine. *Med Teach*. 2012;34(12):e813–e819.

72. Boudreau JD, Liben S, Fuks A. A faculty development workshop in narrative-based reflective writing. *Perspect Med Educ*. 2012;1(3):143–154.

73. *Cambridge Online Dictionary*. Cambridge: Cambridge University Press; 2017.

74. Epner DE, Baile WF. Difficult conversations: teaching medical oncology trainees communication skills one hour at a time. *Acad Med*. 2014;89(4):578.

75. Kuper A. Literature and medicine: a problem of assessment. *Acad Med*. 2006;81(10):S128–S137.

76. Learman LA, Autry AM, O'Sullivan P. Reliability and validity of reflection exercises for obstetrics and gynecology residents. *Am J Obstet Gynecol*. 2008;198(4):461.

77. Kidd MG, Connor JT. Striving to do good things: teaching humanities in Canadian medical schools. *J Med Humanit*. 2008;29(1):45–54.

78. Bleakley A, Marshall R. Can the science of communication inform the art of the medical humanities? *Med Educ*. 2013;47(2):126–133.

79. Bleakley A. *Medical Humanities and Medical Education: How the Medical Humanities Can Shape Better Doctors*. Oxon: Routledge; 2015.

80. Ousager J, Johannessen H. Humanities in undergraduate medical education: a literature review. *Acad Med*. 2010;85(6):988–998.

81. Perry M, Maffulli N, Willson S, Morrissey D. The effectiveness of arts-based interventions in medical education: a literature review. *Med Educ*. 2011;45(2):141–148.

82. Hurwitz B. Medical humanities: lineage, excursionary sketch and rationale. *J Med Ethics*. 2013;39(11):672–674.

83. Schwartz AW, Abramson JS, Wojnowich I, Accordino R, Ronan EJ, Rifkin MR. Evaluating the impact of the humanities in medical education. *Mt Sinai J Med*. 2009;76(4):372–380.

84. Worly B. Professionalism education of OB/GYN resident physicians: What makes a difference? *Open J Obstet Gynecol*. 2013;3(1):137.

85. Charon R. Commentary: calculating the contributions of humanities to medical practice—motives, methods, and metrics. *Acad Med*. 2010;85(6):935–937.

86. Belling C. Commentary: sharper instruments: on defending the humanities in undergraduate medical education. *Acad Med*. 2010;85(6):938–940.

87. Polianski IJ, Fangerau H. Toward "harder" medical humanities: moving beyond the "two cultures" dichotomy. *Acad Med*. 2012;87(1):121–126.

88. Pattison S. Medical humanities: a vision and some cautionary notes. *Med Humanit*. 2003;29(1):33–36.

89. Kuper A, Whitehead C, Hodges BD. Looking back to move forward: using history, discourse and text in medical education research: AMEE Guide No. 73. *Med Teach*. 2013;35(1):e849–e860.

90. Dennhardt S, Apramian T, Lingard L, Torabi N, Arntfield S. Rethinking research in the medical humanities: a scoping review and narrative synthesis of quantitative outcome studies. *Med Educ*. 2016;50(3):285–299.

91. Freire P. *Pedagogy of the Oppressed.* New York: Bloomsbury; 2000.

92. Reis SP, Wald HS, Monroe AD, Borkan JM. Begin the BEGAN (The Brown Educational Guide to the Analysis of Narrative)— A framework for enhancing educational impact of faculty feedback to students' reflective writing. *Patient Educ Couns.* 2010;80(2):253–259.

93. Wald HS, Borkan JM, Taylor JS, Anthony D, Reis SP. Fostering and evaluating reflective capacity in medical education: developing the REFLECT rubric for assessing reflective writing. *Acad Med.* 2012;87(1):41–50.

94. Miller-Kuhlmann R, O'Sullivan PS, Aronson L. Essential steps in developing best practices to assess reflective skill: a comparison of two rubrics. *Med Teach.* 2016;38(1):75–81.

95. O'Sullivan P, Aronson L, Chittenden E, Niehaus B, Learman L. Reflective ability rubric and user guide. *MedEdPortal.* 2010;Aug 26.

96. Charon R, Hermann MN. A sense of story, or why teach reflective writing? *Acad Med.* 2012;87(1):5.

97. Moniz T, Arntfield S, Miller K, Lingard L, Watling C, Regehr G. Considerations in the use of reflective writing for student assessment: issues of reliability and validity. *Med Educ.* 2015;49(9):901–908.

98. Ogdie AR, Reilly JB, Pang WG, et al. RIME: Reflections on performance—seen through their eyes: residents' reflections on the cognitive and contextual components of diagnostic errors in medicine. *Acad Med.* 2012;87(10):1361.

99. Moon M, Taylor HA, McDonald EL, Hughes MT, Beach MC, Carrese JA. Analyzing reflective narratives to assess the ethical reasoning of pediatric residents. *Narrat Inq Bioeth.* 2013;3(2):165–174.

100. Sim K, Sum MY, Navedo D. Use of narratives to enhance learning of research ethics in residents and researchers. *BMC Med Educ.* 2015;15(1):41.

101. Hoffman LA, Shew RL, Vu TR, Brokaw JJ, Frankel RM. Is reflective ability associated with professionalism lapses during medical school? *Acad Med.* 2016;91(6):853–857.

4

"Learning on the Job"

Ethics in Postgraduate Medical Education

CHRYSSA McALISTER, MONA GUPTA,

CARRIE BERNARD, NEDA GHIAM,

AND PHILIP C. HÉBERT

"I'm always ready to learn, although I do not always like being taught."

—WINSTON CHURCHILL[a]

Introduction

In this chapter we briefly review the evolution of ethics[b] as a pedagogical component of postgraduate medical education (PGME). Fundamentally, medical ethics is not about ensuring trainees have the right answers. It is about encouraging self-reflection and an awareness of alternatives. We consider four areas of specialization— family medicine, psychiatry, surgery, and pediatrics—to illustrate current standards and future directions in postgraduate (PG) ethics training.

---

a. Thanks to Dr. Jonathan Hellman for this quote.

b. In this chapter, "ethics" is used interchangeably with "morality," "medical ethics," and "bioethics."

The Evolution of Postgraduate Training

Beginning in the 1960s, commentators on medicine observed there were issues and dilemmas raised by medical science to which it did not, and could not, have the answers. Advances in medicine, especially in intensive care unit (ICU) care and failing organ replacement, made real, effective options available to perilously ill patients. The unique challenge of modern medicine was whether and how patient values, wishes, and beliefs were to be taken into account in making decisions about such options. A genuine interest in the patient's well-being has long been important for physicians. But a new emphasis in ethics and law upon patient autonomy—and the cognate notions of informed consent, capacity, and confidentiality—radically transformed the doctor-patient relationship.[1]

It was in this context of transformative medicine that a number of high-level reports from American presidential commissions on research,[2] end-of-life care,[3] and consent[4] were released in the late 1970s and early 1980s. The reports rested on four basic principles of bioethics—patient autonomy, justice, beneficence, and nonmaleficence—to be used in good decision-making in medicine and medical research ("principlism"). These reports and the principles they used were extremely influential and were widely adopted by physicians, philosophers, and medical educators.[5]

The "principlist" approach to ethics is not without its critics.[6] Of concern with principlism is its relative inattention to the development of moral character and its tendency to lapse into an algorithmic, mechanical style of decision-making. The dominant ethical paradigms are deontological (duty-based, Kantian-type) theories or consequentialist (utilitarian outcome-based) theories. Happiness or capability theories, narrative ethics, virtue theory, feminist ethics, and casuistry are chief among ethical approaches that are rivals to, or completions of, the dominant ethical paradigms. Thus, capability theories spell out what should be the proper consequences of moral action. Virtue theory, by contrast, suggests that there are certain characteristics of the "good clinician" that are intrinsically good. Most approaches to modern medical ethics are, however, hybrid theories—combining duty-based and outcome-based elements. (See Box 4.1; note this list is far from exhaustive.)

Happiness or capability theories propose that the goal of ethical acts is to maximize the happiness or the capabilities (such as freedom to choose) of individuals. Narrative ethics calls for thick descriptions of cases encouraging greater input from the patient and the care provider. This approach is readily familiar to clinicians used to writing up luminous case descriptions. Narrative ethics also looks to reading fiction as a better way of encouraging moral development. Likewise, virtue theory emphasizes the personal aspect of medicine and asks: What would a "good doctor" do? It considers traits such as altruism, honesty, and trustworthiness to be good in themselves and to be more surefooted guides to right action. Indeed, a keen sense of intuition and clinical discernment in deciding what to do seems necessary to the practice of the art of good medical care. Feminist theory considers how men and women may approach ethical issues differently and emphasizes caring

---

BOX 4.1 A Typology of Some Ethical Theories

1. Consequentialism
    a. Utilitarianism
    b. Happiness or capability theories
2. Deontology
    a. Kantian theory
    b. Virtue theory
3. Hybrid theories
    a. Principlism
    b. Narrative ethics
    c. Feminism
    d. Casuistry

relationships and responsibilities rather than more abstract rights and duties of moral agents. Finally, casuistry—long derided as sophistical excuse making—has recently been revived as a form of reasoning from cases that eschews principles in favor of paradigms or analogies by which different cases can be compared and contrasted.

All of these approaches to ethics are fruitful. It is unlikely that the differences between them will ever be eliminated. Each is a perspective on ethics and right action that provides something unique and important.[7] Moreover, the disputes between them do not have to be resolved in order for ethics to be clinically useful or to be taught. It is notable, for example, that two authors, who diverged on the level of grand ethical theory (deontology vs. consequentialism), could still agree on concrete, everyday ethical issues and wrote the most well-known textbook on bioethics, *Principles of Biomedical Ethics*.[8] The requirement for modern ethics teaching is not consistency in ethical theory but pragmatism, thoughtfulness, and reflection. This may be why much theoretical content is not pertinent to medical training and why elaborating lists of "essential" topics in ethics is often otiose (although useful as a starting point). The key to success to teaching ethics is not so much finding the "what" to teach but discovering the "how" to teach. Like Churchill, residents always want to learn; they just don't want to be taught ethics in the same way that other medical content areas are taught. Ethics as a pedagogical tool requires attention to fostering moral thoughtfulness and moral concern, not the inculcation of the "right" answers. How we should help our trainees learn ethics is through the use and mentoring of illuminating cases—the kind of cases that captured our interest and motivated many of us to do work in ethics.

In response to movements during the 1960s and 1970s favoring patient self-determination, medical schools had already begun revamping their teaching in ethics. From a simple reliance on imparting norms of professional courtesy and duty-based ethics credos, programs began to incorporate more critical teaching of modern bioethics and professionalism into *undergraduate* medical education,[9,10] but it was recognized that ethical attitudes and ethical sensitivity of undergraduate medical trainees degraded over time.[11]

Many now view residency as the ideal time for ethics education.[12] Residents hold increasing responsibilities for the care of patients and must make difficult decisions. The recognition of the "hidden curriculum" and its powerful impact on the formative (and sometimes less than ethically appropriate) attitudes, beliefs, and practices of trainees suggests that residency programs must develop protective, positive responses for their trainees.[13] The opportunity and need to shore up ethics teaching—ensuring appropriate core values, behaviors, and attitudes of medicine are encouraged—in PG training is part of that protective response.

The teaching of ethics during PG training is distinct from undergraduate ethics instruction. Undergraduate ethics teaching needs to be general—the successful medical school graduate need only be familiar with a broad scope of ethical knowledge in order to cope with medicine in a supervised setting. As a resident, however, he or she will be gradually introduced to more and more independence in practice. Independence in practice means that residents have to develop the ability, among other things, to recognize and identify the ethical aspects of care and make difficult ethical decisions, especially in their area of specialization. The ethical and professional knowledge and skills to be learned will be, to some extent, specific to a training program. All trainees will benefit from having familiarity with basic ethical principles and a way of reflecting on ethical problems. For some trainees a working knowledge of certain ethical ideas will do and others will require an in-depth knowledge of the same topics. For example, primary care providers or family physicians will need some knowledge of capacity assessment but psychiatrists will need a deeper understanding of it. Furthermore, it is a challenge for faculty to parse an ethical syllabus for learners into the various stages of the curricula.[c]

In 2004, the Accreditation Council for Graduate Medical Education (ACGME) released its Outcome Project (see Box 4.2),[14]

---

c. Breen K. Personal communication. The Australian Medical Council has done so for four of the major colleges (surgery, internal medicine, family medicine, and ICU medicine).

BOX 4.2 Six General Competencies

1. Patient care
2. Medical Knowledge
3. Professionalism
4. Systems-based Practice
5. Practice-based Learning
6. Interpersonal and Communication Skills

Adapted from Swing and the Accreditation Council for Graduate Medical Education.[16]

Advancing Education in Medical Professionalism, a project initiated in 1998 to improve residents' skills in providing high-quality care to patients. Its purpose was to provide "educational resources for program directors and other medical educators to aid teaching and assessing professionalism, one of the six ACGME general competencies."[15] (See Box 4.2.) Note that bioethics is not a separate competency but is melded in with other competencies.

In 2006 Goold and Stern had observed that, "[d]espite consensus for the idea of training in ethics and professionalism, concrete recommendations about content and evaluation methods are sparse for graduate medical education."[16] A 2014 survey revealed ethics was included in the core curriculum of only 50% of obstetrics-gynecology residency programs, usually taught in an unstructured manner. Of those programs offering ethics teaching, only 43% dedicated five or more hours per year to this topic.[17] But the *quality* of ethics instruction may be more important than the *quantity* of hours of ethics instruction in enabling the self-reflection and thoughtfulness that is critical to moral deliberation.

It has sometimes been argued that ethics and professionalism should be seen as distinct enterprises.[18] Professionalism was traditionally confined to concerns with proper behavior, self- regulation, and avoiding misconduct. By contrast ethics, arguably, has been directed at something broader,[19] a self-reflective and thoughtful exercise as to what one should ideally do in difficult circumstances. But this divide is artificial. In part what can be recommended, as ethical practice, ought to take professional norms into account. Norms and regulations are, like laws, part of the moral landscape. And professionalism, which must consider matters such as the communication skills and the comportment befitting a physician, is profoundly dependent on ethics, on what is required for right and wrong decision-making.

An influential pan-Canadian competency-based report for providing "high quality safe patient care" (Canadian Medical Education Directions for Specialists [CanMEDS])—was released in 2005 (see Figure 4.1)[20] and updated in 2015.[21] It has since been adopted by the

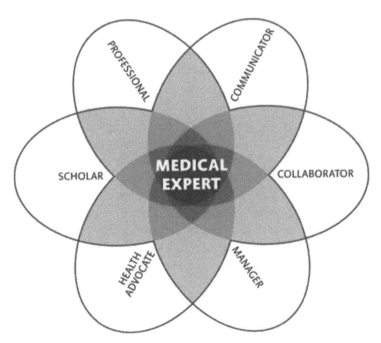

FIGURE 4.1. The CanMEDS role framework.

Royal College of Physicians and Surgeons of Canada, the College of Family Physicians of Canada,[22] the General Medical Council for the United Kingdom,[23] and the Australian Medical Council.[24]

"Competency-based frameworks outline the core knowledge and skills that individual physicians are expected to maintain."[25] Competency-based assessments offer tangible educational objectives by examining candidates to determine if they have the knowledge, attitudes, and skills appropriate for their level of training. They have become standard for PGME programs in medicine. But can bioethics be evaluated in the same way? The answer to this question should be yes, at least partly so, but just how is not a settled question. It depends on the goals and expectations regarding PG ethics teaching.

There have been "successful" ethics PG teaching programs. One center reported on their experience in internal medicine. In a "safe" forum of two-hour small-group sessions led by fellows, residents brought their most difficult cases. The measures of success were that residents "remained engaged" and that "clinically relevant thinking and learning"[26] was facilitated.

The San Antonio Uniformed Services Health Education Consortium observed that, using traditional didactic teaching, "residents had a difficult time recognizing ethical dilemmas."[27] To address this issue, a pragmatic tool for assessing and resolving ethical issues and dilemmas across the hospital was developed. This tool (see Appendices 1 and 2), was "surprisingly helpful" and "100% of program directors . . . would train residents to utilize the tool prior to the arrival of next year's intern class." Success here was defined as the usefulness of the tool to residents and physicians in helping to identify and resolve difficult problems.

Decision tools for managing ethical issues are increasingly popular as ways of helping trainees to recognize and to resolve ethical issues at the PG level. They are meant to ensure that an approach to an ethical dilemma is careful, structured, and holistic. The tool summarized in Box 4.3 has been evaluated and has demonstrated

---

BOX 4.3 An Eight-Step Approach to Ethical Dilemmas:
A Decision Tool

1. Gather all the relevant data as they relate to the case.
2. Identify the basic principles involved and explain their relevance.
3. Consider whether the principles conflict and assess their uncertainty.
4. Formulate a question reflecting the conflict.
5. Decide which principle takes priority, provide rationale, or find an alternative solution for avoiding the conflict.
6. If uncertainty persists, consider what information might be missing that would reduce the uncertainty.
7. Evaluate your decision by asking if it is what a consensus of exemplary doctors would do.
8. Plan practical steps to be taken and future issues that can be foreseen.

Adapted from *The Belmont Report*[3] and Myer et al.[29] See also Appendices 1 and 2.

---

some hopeful results: 84% of residents found it "clarified the ethical concepts in the case" and 83% thought it would be useful "in future interactions with the patient or family."[28]

Residency programs have addressed deficiencies in their practices regarding advance directives,[29] error disclosure,[30] communication,[31] professionalism,[32] and the wise use of medical resources.[33] A positive, proactive ethics PG education should also include less commonly taught matters, such as the physician as patient,[34] coping with difficult patients, physician addiction,[35] sexual or racial harassment,[36] and medical trainee distress and burnout.[37]

These less commonly addressed issues loom large for residents and are often a source of serious moral distress. A simplistic reliance on a decision procedure may fail to do justice to them. Box 4.4 provides 10 simple recommendations for ways to develop PG ethics teaching.

The presupposition is that such initiatives, in addressing and improving ethical reasoning abilities and communication skills,

---

BOX 4.4 10 Core Requirements for PGME Ethics

1. Concentrate on issues and practical cases of importance and relevance to residents.
2. Look to the relevant peer groups, disciplines, and colleges to decide what constitutes comprehensive discipline-specific training—the topics for which residents, to be competent in their field of training, must have an in-depth knowledge of (e.g., medical assistance in dying in geriatrics, confidentiality in psychiatry, consent in surgery, boundary issues/improper conduct in primary care) and the topics for with which they need only be familiar or of which to have a working knowledge.
3. Provide for faculty development.
4. Encourage residents to bring forward their own examples of ethically challenging situations during formal instruction.
5. Use an ethics decision-making tool.
6. Promote self-directed learning and use of online resources.
7. Devote some journal clubs to ethics.
8. Involve residents with skilled mentors in teaching ethics to students or more junior residents.
9. Consider co-teaching sessions with ethicists.
10. Incorporate ethics teaching into the clinic and the regular cycle of rounds and seminars.

can aid in the formation of the attributes of the good clinician—prudent, honest, altruistic, and trustworthy—but there is, admittedly, little empirical evidence to support this claim. Whether such initiatives, if successful, will support and encourage an even more expansive notion of moral sensitivity on the part of medical trainees—the development of moral awareness and discernment—that some would see as the better and bigger target of PGME ethics education is a more challenging question.

Residency programs must craft field-specific cases and issues. To this end they might consider the many useful ethics resources online. A well-maintained online American resource in ethics may be found at the Virtual Mentor site of *JAMA*. This site provides a wealth of salient cases going back to 2010; each case is accompanied by thoughtful responses from a variety of clinicians.[38] The Royal College of Physicians and Surgeons of Canada (RCPSC) maintains an equally broad bank of ethics cases accompanied by discussion of the relevant issues[39] as does the College of Family Physicians of Canada (CFPC).[40] The General Medical Council of the United Kingdom also has a very comprehensive collection of interactive case studies.[41] There is no available data as to whether these excellent resources are used by residents or by PG programs.

It should not be thought that ethics and professionalism teaching must depend on clinical faculty alone. Hospitals have bioethicists or bioethics departments that can help improve the ethical capacity of clinicians. Ethicists can not only bring to bear independent expertise to a clinical problem, but they can also, being familiar with medical jurisprudence and prior cases, be extremely helpful in acting as educators and consultants on ethical issues generally. However, ethicists, who are not clinicians, should not entirely replace the pedagogical role of medical faculty.[42] Their most important role, perhaps, may be to "teach the teachers," so that clinicians, no matter what their background, will feel more comfortable in teaching ethics and professionalism.

We next examine four domains of medicine and provide some suggestions for going forward in these areas.

Postgraduate Family Medicine

PG teachers in departments of family medicine are expected to teach their residents about medical ethics and how to apply their ethics learning to clinical situations as they transition into independent practice. Indeed, the CFPC, the American Academy of Family Physicians, the Royal College of General Practitioners in the United Kingdom, and the Royal College of General Practitioners in Australia all include learning objectives relating to ethics as essential components of PG family medicine programs.[43,44,45,46]

Recent surveys of PG family medicine programs in Canada and the United States revealed considerable variation in time spent teaching about ethics, ethics content, delivery, and evaluation methods. Common topics that could and should be addressed in PG family medicine—and indeed in other residency programs—may be found in Box 4.5. It must be said that, even when ethics teaching

---

BOX 4.5 Top 10 Ethics Topics To Be Addressed

1. Review of medical ethics principles (e.g., autonomy, justice, beneficence, non-malfeasance)
2. Ethical reasoning/analysis as a way to approach ethical dilemmas in clinical practice
3. Consent
4. Confidentiality
5. End-of-life care
6. Conflicts of interest in clinical practice
7. Professional codes of ethics
8. Legal and regulatory aspects of clinical medicine
9. Improper physician conduct
10. Ethical principles relating to medical research

is prioritized, formal assessments of the effectiveness of PG ethics teaching are rare.[47,48]

Some studies (one with neurology residents, one in internal medicine, and one in family medicine) found benefit of a specific ethics curriculum, but none had a comparator group.[49,50,51] More recent evaluations of PG ethics teaching have been limited to resident confidence and preference of teaching styles.[52] Ethics at times seems to be intangible, requiring not just up-to-date knowledge but also awareness of one's own, as well as the others', values and attitudes—its many facets make it a challenge to sort out and measure.

The literature provides no clear guidance regarding best practices for ethics teaching and evaluation in PG family medicine. There are, however, some themes relating to what experts and residents believe might be most useful. Not surprisingly, small-group case-based discussion is preferred to didactic lectures.[53,54] There is also a preference for having ethics teaching integrated with clinical work.[55] These findings are not unique to family medicine, with other specialty residents also describing a preference for case-based teaching integrated into the flow of clinical work.[56]

The literature does provide some direction regarding the challenges educators face when attempting to deliver material relating to ethics in the family medicine residency context with the major barriers being time constraints and lack of faculty confidence in delivering ethics teaching.[57,58] It is essential, therefore, to provide teaching and support to clinical teachers who work with family medicine residents daily in clinic to better facilitate ethics learning relating to real clinical scenarios. As residents will vary in their knowledge and comfort regarding ethical issues, it can be helpful to undertake a needs analysis at the onset of residency. Educators should also look to issues considered critical by hospital authorities, health insurers, and medical regulators. At the top of everyone's list is a program that emphasizes communication,

BOX 4.6 Eight Ways to Develop or Enhance a PG Ethics Curriculum

1. Most importantly, decide on the objectives of the ethics curriculum.
2. Set reasonable expectations. In other words, when initiating an ethics program, avoid being overly ambitious. Focus on a few outstanding issues in depth.
3. At a minimum, ensure residents are familiar with the ethical norms in their fields as articulated in regulatory guidance, hospital policy, university policy, as well as ensure that residents know how and who to access if they need help in ethically difficult situations.
4. Focus on identifying and nurturing ethical sensitivity, increasing awareness of choice, and the need for self-reflection.
5. Integrate ethics into general clinical teaching as much as possible rather than only having stand-alone "ethics sessions."
6. Have sessions devoted to collateral competencies such as improved communication skills, alternate dispute resolution, critical skills, and interprofessional collaborative decision-making.
7. Provide more advanced house staff with opportunities to participate in teaching ethics to more junior learners, such as medical students. As some residents will be themselves untutored in ethics and so unprepared to teach it, they should be paired with an ethicist or an experienced clinician (even ready-to-teach residents can benefit from such co-teaching). This is "learning on the job," not "see one, do one."
8. Encourage clinical faculty to develop their skills and confidence in the delivery of an ethics curriculum by providing them with preprepared seminar notes and pairing them with ethicists, more experienced clinicians, or other knowledgeable faculty (such as lawyers with medical jurisprudence training).

listening, and honesty. A successful PG ethics program will combine practical approaches to issues that are important for the skilled MD. Box 4.6 provides some tips for developing ethics in residency programs generally.

Postgraduate Psychiatry

In a recent article Wada and colleagues note that "'psychiatry residents' ethics education is still an underdeveloped area without consensus regarding the goal(s), content, method, and evaluation of outcomes."[59] Thus, any guidance on how to initiate, implement, and evaluate ethics education in psychiatry will necessarily be preliminary. This section will discuss the relevant published literature in order to illustrate the uncertainty in these domains and will conclude by suggesting certain key issues that programs should consider in constructing their own ethics educational initiatives.

What are the goals of ethics education in PG psychiatry training? Bloch and Green[60] point out that there are several possible answers to this question that can be easily conflated. They note that until recently ethics education has been understood variously as "promoting moral character; developing skills in moral reasoning; moral consciousness-raising; and becoming familiar with what the psychiatric profession regards as desirable ethical norms."

As the movement toward competency-based education has taken hold, specialty-training organizations increasingly view the goal of ethics education as "competence in ethics." Yet, there is no shared understanding of this goal. Variations between countries can lead to important differences in training and, ultimately, in practice. For example, the US ACGME requires that a competent psychiatry resident can recognize "ethical issues in practice and is able to discuss, analyze, and manage these in common clinical situations."[61]

In the UK, the Royal College of Psychiatrists upholds the more modest requirement that trainees adhere to existing ethical codes.[62] The latter goal involves ethics only to the extent that trainees understand there are certain positions in ethics that have already been worked out and agreed upon. The task for trainees is to be aware of them and conform in their behavior. For its part, the RCPSC wishes to ensure that psychiatrists exhibit appropriate professional behaviors in practice: honesty, integrity, commitment, compassion, respect, and altruism (although these are described as behaviors, they are in fact virtues); demonstrate a commitment to delivering the highest quality care and maintenance of competence; and recognize and appropriately respond to ethical issues encountered in psychiatry.[63]

Within these conceptions of "competence," there is room still for individual programs to determine which aspects of Bloch and Green's schema they want and are able to emphasize. Establishing the goal(s) of an ethics curriculum is thus a crucial first step for any program, as it is the goals that determine the content, method, and outcomes for evaluation.

Several authors provide lists of topics that could be addressed or that residents and faculty believe should be addressed in a formal ethics curriculum.[64,65,66,67] Many such topics revolve around questions that are already subject to legislation. On the one hand, this may reflect the fact that certain psychiatric practices, such as involuntary hospitalization, operate within a legislative framework. The need to apply the law in specific clinical cases is a natural pressure point where ethical questions or dilemmas may arise.

On the other hand, anchoring ethics teaching in medico-legal domains can give the impression that ethical problems in the clinic can be resolved by recourse to the law when, in fact, it is precisely the complexity of real-life cases that resists easy resolution by way of a legal test or standard. Is there pedagogical value in discussing these ethical issues outside the real clinical context in which they occur in a stand-alone ethics curriculum? This remains an unsettled question. But because specialty-training organizations require that psychiatry residents receive a minimum level of training, program directors would be right to worry about having no dedicated ethics curriculum or simply leaving such instruction to the discretion of individual supervisors.

Gupta et al,[68] as well as Hoop,[69] point out that offering a formal curriculum in ethics must be complemented by attention to the hidden curriculum in ethics which may offer content that is at odds with, or even directly contradictory to, the objectives of the formal curriculum. Indeed, the Health Canada–funded *Future of Medical Education Postgraduate Project* report[70] recommended that counterproductive elements of the hidden curriculum be addressed within PG training programs. However, this has yet to find its way into the suggestions for curricular content discussed in the literature. This omission may reflect the fact that the hidden curriculum lies embedded within the cultural practices of organizations (e.g., training programs, hospitals). Addressing it will have to involve those with the power to incite organizational change rather than through a curriculum directed to residents alone.

Dingle et al. offer a lengthy inventory of possible approaches to the development of ethical reasoning.[71,72] Some authors have gone a step further, attempting to evaluate a specific approach or curriculum. For example, Wada et al. evaluated a one-day workshop offered to psychiatry residents whose outcomes were to improve knowledge of ethics including the ability to identify ethics issues and to apply ethical theories to reach solutions.[73] They concluded that such a workshop could achieve these outcomes. Meanwhile Green and colleagues[74] also offered a one-day workshop whose objective was to influence participants' ethical sensitivity. Using a specific measurement tool to assess this change, they demonstrated that ethical sensitivity increased immediately following the workshop although they acknowledged that they could not predict the duration of the effect.

In light of the lack of consensus surrounding the goals and content of ethics education in psychiatry, as well as the uncertainty regarding optimal pedagogical methods, how can programs construct a curriculum for their residents that will, at the least, meet accreditation standards?

Agreeing upon the goals of an ethics curriculum is a necessary first step. The reality of the time constraints, lack of background knowledge of ethics amongst the majority of residents, and absence of qualified teachers suggests that modest goals are in order. These might include ensuring that residents are aware of ethical norms and the behaviors that demonstrate respect for those norms and that they can identify ethically challenging situations and know how to access assistance when needed. Such practical goals align with the need within a competency-based education framework to assess outcomes of learning. Ensuring that residents are aware of existing ethical norms and that they demonstrate appropriate behaviors are learning outcomes that are feasible to capture.

While time, resources, and the requirements of specialty training organizations will necessarily steer programs toward pragmatic aims in their educational offerings, an ethics curriculum in psychiatry cannot ignore the fundamental philosophical debates that continue to surround the field. These include the nature of mind and mental illness, the distinction between normal and abnormal, and the appropriate aims of psychiatric treatment. Ultimately, all ethical problems in psychiatry stem from the basic idea that there is a legitimate diversity of views about what constitutes good mental health. This core concept is an essential starting point for the content of an ethics curriculum for PG psychiatry.

Postgraduate Surgery

Surgical residency programs have historically taught relevant ethics principles and concepts to trainees through an apprenticeship model of applied ethics. Surgeons frequently guide patients and their families through complex decision-making and informed consent, break bad news, and deal with palliation and end-of-life care. Surgeons work as fiduciaries in their daily practice and understand the importance of trust in the patient-physician relationship.

Although exposure to key ethical concepts is common through this historical model, formalized ethics education provides more comprehensive exposure to ethics principles and develops the necessary tools to resolve ethical dilemmas appropriately, with inclusion of societal and institutional ethical concepts that may not arise in daily practice.[75] Canadian surgical residency training programs today are mandated by the RCPSC to have formal specialty-specific ethics education. Despite this requirement, a survey of ethics coordinators across surgical programs suggests a wide variation in content, timing and methodology.[76] Similarly, ethics education is included in the majority of PG surgical training programs in the United States[77] with the content and volume of ethics teaching activities often dependent on the presence of a faculty member with a special interest in ethics teaching[78].

The majority of Canadian surgical trainees, with the exception of ophthalmology and obstetrics and gynecology, write the mandatory RPCSC Principles of Surgery (POS) examination after two years of residency training. At the University of Toronto, trainees receive eight 1.5-hour ethics sessions as part of the POS lecture series the content of which is based on the RCPSC bioethics curriculum. Topics on the RCPSC website cover a broad range of subjects and include primers on conflict resolution, legal concepts, and fundamental bioethics principles.[79] As yet there has been no evaluation on the effectiveness of the ethics curricula.

Many surgical programs at the University of Toronto teach ethics concepts through case-based discussions, according to the 2012 qualitative study by Howard et al.[86] Case-based content allows trainees to use concrete examples and develop a better understanding of the complexity often present in philosophical ethics arguments. Narrative writing can also enhance ethics teaching in surgery by providing vivid scenarios that evoke empathy and compassion and engage the trainee in discussion.[80,81] Other formats for ethics teaching reported include journal clubs, role-playing, standardized patients, and debate. Teaching methods and ethics content were selected based on coordinator experiences, consultation with other faculty and trainees, consultation with ethics experts, and consideration of current ethical issues discussed in the media.

Ophthalmology surgical training programs across Canada send residents every two years to the Halifax Ethics Symposium in Ophthalmology.[82] This two-day conference covers a variety of relevant ophthalmology ethics topics with didactic sessions followed by small-group discussions. The curriculum is designed for resident trainees with content delivered by guest speakers and local faculty and is a simple and effective way for PG programs to incorporate relevant ethics teaching into the curriculum without acquiring local ethics resources and expertise.

Surgical programs may also choose to incorporate more intensive ethics training into their local curriculum. The University of Toronto Department of Ophthalmology and Vision Sciences developed an ethics and CanMEDS curriculum in 2015 to ensure comprehensive skills development in core competencies. The curriculum is delivered over four half-days and one evening journal club, with resource papers given to students and tutor-guides developed to allow the content to be delivered by any faculty member. See Table 4.1.

The success of the overall curriculum relies on the concept that included content addresses issues relevant to current trainees and also to current practicing ophthalmologists. Multiple teaching styles are utilized with a focus on case-based interactive discussions that allow trainees to reflect on their own experiences. Every two years trainee input into topics are solicited and included in an anonymized collection and the curriculum in the subsequent two-year cycle can be modified accordingly. Trainees also have an opportunity to provide feedback through an evaluation form given at the beginning and the end of the teaching cycle.

Resources for surgical trainees in bioethics include the bioethics content on the websites for both the RCPSC and the American College of Surgeons (ACS). RCPSC has online tools for physicians and trainees to use with 47 ethics cases, five primers, and 10 interactive modules. The Association of Professors of Obstetrics and Gynecology, which represents both American and Canadian obstetrical and gynecological surgeons, has an ethics case study available

TABLE 4.1 A Surgical Residency Ethics Curriculum in Five Half-Days

	Teaching Method	Resources
Session 1: Professionalism	Student-centered open-ended discussion followed by tutor-led case-based discussion	Practice Guide: Medical Professionalism and College Policies[105]
Session 2: Fundamental Concepts in Bioethics	Small-group case-based session on three ethics scenarios	Introduction to an ethical decision-making framework Tutor guide with core ethical principles and values Peer-review paper handouts on breaking bad news, mandatory reporting, and truth-telling
Session 3: Innovation, Research and Conflicts of Interest (COI)	Journal club evening discussion on innovations in surgery and COI Informal discussion on trainee experience with industry and methods to address and resolve COI	Relevant journal articles preassigned Tutor guide with highlighted features on how articles should be critically appraised to identify COI Identifies how COI impact different stages of research Discussion of disclosure policies for journals Discussion on the adoption of innovations into practice and relevant COI

(continued)

TABLE 4.1 Continued

	Teaching Method	Resources
Session 4: Combining Insured and Uninsured Services	Small-group tutor-led discussion followed by debate Students assigned into two groups to defend different viewpoints and highlight the complexity of the scenario Didactic presentation on the combining of insured and non-insured surgical services	Newspaper and popular media handouts with a scripted scenario Peer-review paper on combining insured and non-insured services given to students Tutor guide with highlighted ethical values and principles relevant to case
Session 5: Truth-Telling and Disclosure	Student-led discussion on trainee participation in surgery Tutor-led discussion/a reading of peer-review literature on informed consent for trainee participation in surgery	Scripted scenario on deception surrounding trainee participation to elicit discussion Tutor guide highlights ethical terms to review including fiduciary duty, respect for persons, autonomy, informed consent, beneficence and non-maleficence.

online.[83] The Royal College of Surgeons in the United Kingdom has online e-learning modules on consent and ethics; a comprehensive guide to Good Surgical Practice; podcasts on the legal, ethical, and professional considerations in informed consent; and an e-learning module on the importance of candor in maintaining patient trust.[84] The ACS has two volumes available, one on ethical issues in clinical surgery for practicing surgeons and one for trainees, along with a continuing medical education knowledge assessment.[85]

Formalized evaluation of trainee understanding and application of ethics principles remains a challenge in PG surgical training programs. Evaluations reported in the literature suggest that surgical trainees score poorly on formal assessments of ethics knowledge,[86] which may represent an ethics knowledge deficit or alternatively may suggest a difficulty in formally assessing ethics knowledge through traditional evaluation tools.

Despite the challenge faced in testing surgical ethics knowledge in PG trainees, evaluation remains an essential component in the development of robust surgical ethics curricula. Appropriate evaluation— yet to be validated—will both ensure that trainees acquire the necessary ethics knowledge and skills and also that the ethics curriculum is effectively delivering the necessary material to trainees.

Postgraduate Pediatrics

The ethical practice of pediatrics, similar to other specialties, requires competency in professionalism through the development of a "professional identity." Residents are expected to develop their moral character and attitudes as virtuous ethical professionals as part of learning the clinical skills to care for patients.[87]

The unique nature of pediatrics as a medical specialty is an important contextual factor in teaching ethical behavior to pediatric PG trainees. PG trainees require a specialized skillset to address the unique ethical scenarios facing pediatricians. They must learn how to balance their legitimate advocacy for neonates and children, who cannot speak for themselves, and the liberty interests of parents to raise their offspring as they see fit. Some parents may be unprepared and feel overwhelmed when facing complex medical issues regarding their children.[88] Pediatricians are also tasked with evaluating and understanding the developing autonomy of the adolescent to determine the level of their competency and the extent of their ability to participate in making medical decisions. The challenges in teaching ethics in pediatrics are related to the unique character of the ethical issues that arise in pediatrics, frequently having to do with addressing power imbalances, maintaining the therapeutic alliance with parents, and distinguishing abuse from suboptimal care.[89]

Ethical teaching is most appropriately embedded in the professional role in competency-based education. In the *Objectives of Residency Training in Pediatrics* by the RCPSC drafted in 2008, ethics is recognized as a fundamental aspect of professionalism.[90] In the 2010 *General Pediatrics Advanced Training Curriculum* by the Royal Australasian College of Physicians, ethics is stated as an explicit learning objective in the curriculum and ethical behavior is an expected outcome for residents upon completion of training.[91] The Pediatrics Milestone Project, a joint initiative of the ACGME and the American Academy of Pediatrics for the evaluation of residents, requires "ethical behavior" as part of professional conduct, considered one of the milestones for pediatric trainees.[92] The most effective method to teach and evaluate the requisite ethical character of physicians, however, remains a challenge for PG pediatrics as it does for other residency programs.

Despite the emphasis on ethics and professionalism, influencing ethical behavior and attitudes remains one of the most complex core contents in medical education.[93] In 1997 the medical ethics faculty at the Children's Hospital in Seattle identified the following obstacles in implementing an ethics curriculum for pediatric residents: time constraints, scheduling difficulties and lack of continuity, negative attitudes of residents toward the material, and inadequate ethics training among faculty.[94] More recently, in 2009, Lang et al. in a survey of the Association of Pediatrics Program Directors (APPD), continued to find that PGME ethics teaching was still often unstructured and that curricular crowding as the main barrier to incorporating ethics and professionalism into the pediatric residency curriculum.[95]

In 2013, Cook et al. surveyed the members of APPD again to see if the changes had occurred given the greater number of resources available to programs. They once more reported crowding in the curriculum followed by lack of faculty expertise, lack of faculty and trainee interest, and lack of administrative support as barriers to develop and maintain ethics and professionalism curricula in the pediatric residency programs.[96] As with other PG programs, consistent and effective methods for teaching and evaluating ethics in pediatrics residency are lacking.[97] The majority of programs teach ethics and professionalism without a structured curriculum and a few still do not provide any such instruction.

Some practices as regards PGME may be recommended (see Box 4.6). Ethics training must focus on encouraging ethical sensitivity and the capacity for self-reflection. This is not easy to achieve. A good place to start in encouraging ethical self-reflection might be to consider the issue of error in medicine. Two outstanding articles are Rick Boyte's article on adverse outcomes in pediatrics[98] and David Hilfiker's early piece on error in family medicine.[99] Both are powerfully written from the erring clinician's perspective. Similar reflective articles may be found in all major medical journals.

The evaluation of ethics and professionalism poses a challenge to residency programs. Should they be evaluated separately or together? In a survey of 96 pediatric residency program directors by Kesselheim et al. in 2012, they expressed only moderate satisfaction with current strategies for evaluating professionalism.[100] In 2014, a study by Rosenbluth et al. showed that, when asked to assess residents, faculty tend to rely on generalized impressions and global behaviors rather than specific behaviors. Traits relating to professionalism were mentioned by 96% of faculty as an important aspect of being "the best resident."[101] However, Warren et al. reported in 2012 that Canadian program directors in the seven largest RCPSC programs including pediatrics find the elements of the professional role difficult to teach and assess.[102] They suggested that evaluating the effectiveness of teaching ethics and professionalism in changing attitudes and behaviors should be a priority in PG programs.

Conclusions

Individual PG programs must fulfill accreditation standards in ethics education as defined by the specialty training body in their own countries. Beyond fulfilling these requirements, which in Canada consists of having some kind of formal ethics education in place, programs must first determine what the goals of ethics education are. Is it to ensure all trainees are fully aware of how to apply or comply with established ethical norms? There is a rich philosophical debate as to whether medical ethics can be truly taught.[103] Ethics is not just one more content area to be mastered—true learning in this area will require attention to encouraging trainee self-reflection.

The goals of PG ethics training will influence the time the program is willing to commit to ethics education, the faculty resources required, the content and pedagogical methods, and the outcomes to be evaluated. It is easier to develop ethical reasoning skills, such as learning to apply an ethics decision procedure (see Box 4.3), than it is to enable the genesis of moral character. While ethics should and will be subject to evaluation of its effectiveness, there is no consensus as to how best to do so, especially as regards the more expansive notion of ethics.

There has been a positive evolution in medical ethics education, interest, and instruction.[104] It is fair to say, however, that despite the enthusiasm for bioethics teaching at the PG level, ethics instruction in residency programs remains haphazard and underevaluated. We all believe it is important, but how important and just how it is to be best taught and evaluated remain unsettled questions.

A sample curriculum to accompany this chapter can be found online at http://cahh.ca/resources/ouplesson-plans/.

References

1. Hébert PC. *Doing Right: A Practical Guide to Ethics for Physicians and Medical Trainees.* 3rd ed. Toronto: Oxford University Press, 2014: 27–34.
2. Office of the Secretary Ethical Principles and Guidelines for the Protection of Human Subjects of Research, National Commission for the Protection of Human Subjects of Biomedical and Behavioural Research. *The Belmont Report.* https://www.hhs.gov/ohrp/regulations-and-policy/belmont-report/. Published April 18, 1979. Accessed March 27, 2017.
3. President's Commission for the Study of Ethical Problems in Medicine and Biomedical and Behavioral Research. *Deciding to Forego Life-Sustaining Treatment.* http://hdl.handle.net/10822/559344. Published March 1983. Accessed March 27, 2017.
4. President's Commission for the Study of Ethical Problems in Medicine and Biomedical and Behavioral Research. *Making Health Care Decisions: A Report on the Ethical and Legal Implications of Informed Consent in the Patient-Practitioner Relationship, Volume One: Report.* https://repository.library.georgetown.edu/handle/10822/559354. Published October 1982. Accessed March 29, 2017.
5. See, for example, Pelčić G. Bioethics and medicine. *Croat Med J.* 2013, 54(1): 1–2. doi:10.3325/cmj.2013.54.1
6. Clouser KD, Gert B. A critique of principlism. *J Med Philos.* 1990; 15(2): 219–236. doi:https://doi.org/10.1093/jmp/15.2.219
7. Wolf S. Hiking the ridge. In: Parfit D. *On What Matters, Volume Two.* Oxford: Oxford University Press; 2011.
8. Beauchamp T, Childress J. *Principles of Biomedical Ethics.* 7th ed. London: Oxford University Press; 2012.
9. Swick H, Szenas P, Danoff D, et al. Education teaching professionalism in undergraduate medical education. *JAMA.* 1999; 282(9): 830–832. doi:10.1001/jama.282.9.830
10. Association of Faculties of Medicine of Canada. *The Future of Medical Education in Canada: A Collective Vision for MD Education.* https://afmc.ca/future-of-medical-education-in-canada/medical-doctor-project/pdf/FMEC_CollectiveVisionMDEducation_EN.compressed.pdf. Published 2010. Accessed December 1, 2016.
11. Goldie J, Schwartz L, McConnachie A, Morrison J. The impact of a modern medical curriculum on students' proposed behaviour

on meeting ethical dilemmas. *Med Educ.* 2004; 38(9): 942–949. doi:10.1111/j.1365-2929.2004.01915

12. Cooke M, Irby DM, O'Brien BC. *Educating Physicians: A Call for Reform of Medical School and Residency.* San Francisco: Jossey-Bass; 2010.

13. Hafferty FW. Beyond curriculum reform: Confronting medicine's hidden curriculum. *Acad Med.* 1998; 73(4): 403–407.

14. Swing RC, Accreditation Council for Graduate Medical Education. The ACGME Outcome Project: retrospective and prospective. *Med Teach.* 2007; 29(7): 648–654. doi:10.1080/01421590701392903

15. ACGME Outcome Project. *Advancing Education in Medical Professionalism.* An Educational Resource from the ACGME Outcome Project. Enhancing residency education through outcomes assessment. https://www.usahealthsystem.com/workfiles/com_docs/gme/2011%20Links/Professionalism%20-%20Faculty%20Dev..pdf. Published 2004. Accessed December 2, 2016.

16. Goold SD, Stern DT. Ethics and professionalism: What does a resident need to learn? *Am J Bioeth.* 2006; 6(4): 9–17. doi:10.1080/15265160600755409

17. Byrne J, Straub H, DiGiovanni L, Chor J. Evaluation of ethics education in obstetrics and gynecology residency programmes. *Am J Obstet Gynecol.* 2015; 212(3): 397:1–8. doi:10.1016/j.ajog.2014.12.027

18. Salloch S. Same same but different: why we should care about the distinction between professionalism and ethics. *BMC Med Ethics.* 2016; 17: 44. doi:10.1186/s12910-016-0128-y

19. Cole P, Block L, Wu A. On higher ground: Ethical reasoning and its relationship with and error disclosure. *BMJ Quality & Safety.* 2013; 22(7): 580–585.

20. Frank J. *The CanMEDs 2005 Physician Competency Framework: Better Standards, Better Physicians, Better Care.* Ottawa: Royal College of Physicians and Surgeons of Canada. http://www.royalcollege.ca/portal/page/portal/rc/common/documents/canmeds/resources/publications/framework_full_e.pdf. Published 2005. Accessed December 1, 2016.

21. Frank JR, Snell L, Sherbino J, eds. *CanMEDS 2015 Physician Competency Framework.* Ottawa: Royal College of Physicians and Surgeons of Canada; 2015. http://canmeds.royalcollege.ca/uploads/en/framework/CanMEDS%202015%20Framework_EN_Reduced.pdf. Accessed July 4, 2017.

22. Busing N. *The Review of PGME in Canada: The Future of Medical Education in Canada. The Postgraduate Project.* http://www.nes.scot.nhs.uk/media/11426/5_Review_of_PGME_in%20Canada_Bursing.pdf. Published May 1, 2012, Accessed November 23, 2016.

23. Kopelman P. The future of UK medical education curriculum—what type of medical graduates do we need? *Fut Hosp J.* 2014; 1(1):41–46. doi:10.7861/futurehosp.14.011

24. Breen K, Cordner S, Thomson C. *Good Medical Practice: Professionalism, Ethics, and Law.* 4th ed. Kingston: Australian Medical Council; 2016.

25. Eva K, et al. Medical Education Assessment Advisory Committee: *Report to the Medical Council of Canada on Current Issues in Health Professional and Health Professional Trainee Assessment.* http://mcc.ca/wp-content/uploads/Reports-MEAAC.pdf. Published April 23, 2013. Accessed January 27, 2017.

26. Vertrees S, Shuman A, Fins J. Learning by doing: Effectively incorporating ethics education into residency training. *J Gen Intern Med.* 2012; 28(4): 578–582. doi:10.1007/s11606-012-2277-0

27. Meyer E, Ford C, Thaxton R, Anders G, Jefferson T, Fruendt J, Harrison S. A pragmatic approach to professional and ethical dilemmas. *J Grad Med Educ.* 2014; 6(2): 357–358. doi:http://dx.doi.org/10.4300/JGME-D-14-00088.1

28. Alfandre D, Rhodes R. Improving ethics education during residency training. *Med Teach.* 2009; 31(6): 513–517. PMID: 19811167

29. Colbert C, et al. Enhancing competency in professionalism: Targeting resident advance directive education. *J Grad Med Educ.* 2010; 2(2): 278–282. doi:10.4300/JGME-D-10-00003.1

30. Martinez W, et al. Role-modeling and medical error disclosure: A national survey of trainees. *Acad Med.* 2014; 89(3): 482–489.

31. Brown S, et al. Radiology trainees' comfort with difficult conversations and attitudes about professionalism: Effect of a communication skills workshop. *J Am Coll Radiol.* 2014;11(8): 781–787 doi:10.1016/j.jacr.2014.01.018

32. Larkin G. Evaluating professionalism in emergency medicine: Clinical ethical competence. *Acad Emerg Med.* 1999; 6(4):302–311.

33. American College of Physicians. *Introduction to Version 3.0 of the High Value Care Curriculum for Internal Medicine Residents.* https://www.acponline.org/clinical-information/high-value-care/medical-educators-resources/curriculum-for-educators-and-residents. Published July 2012. Accessed April 2, 2017.

34. Hébert PC. Thrown for a loop. In: *Good Medicine: The Art of Ethical Care in Canada*. Toronto: Doubleday Canada, 2016: 41–64.

35. Hill AB. Breaking the stigma—a physician's perspective on self-care and recovery. *N Engl J Med*. 2017; 376: 1103–1105. doi:10.1056/NEJMp1615974

36. Koven S. Letter to a young female physician. *N Engl J Med*. 2017; 376: 1907–1909. doi:10.1056/NEJMp1702010

37. Muller D. Kathryn. *N Engl J Med*. 2017; 376:1101–1103. doi:10.1056/NEJMp1615141

38. American Medical Association. AMA Journal of Ethics Archives. http://journalofethics.ama-assn.org/site/archives.html. Accessed November 21, 2016.

39. Royal College of Physicians and Surgeons of Canada. Bioethics. http://www.royalcollege.ca/rcsite/bioethics-e. Accessed January 9, 2017.

40. College of Family Physicians in Canada Ethics Committee. Family Medicine Bioethics Curriculum: Clinical Cases and References. http://www.cfpc.ca/projectassets/templates/re-source.aspx?id=1027&langType=4105. Published 2005. Accessed January 9, 2017.

41. General Medical Council. Good Medical Practice. http://www.gmc-uk.org/guidance/good_medical_practice.asp. Updated April 29, 2014. Accessed March 31, 2017.

42. Siegler M. Lessons from 30 years of teaching clinical ethics. *Virtual Mentor*. 2001; 3(10). http://journalofethics.ama-assn.org/2001/10/medu1-0110.html. Accessed April 1, 2017.

43. Tannenbaum D, Konkin J, Parsons E, Saucier D, Shaw L, Walsh A, Kerr J, Organek A. *CanMEDS-Family Medicine: A Framework of Competencies in Family Medicine*. College of Family Physicians of Canada. http://www.cfpc.ca/ProjectAssets/Templates/Resource.aspx?id=303. Published October 2009. Accessed November 19, 2016.

44. *American Academy of Family Physicians. Recommended Curriculum Guidelines for Family Medicine Residents: Medical Ethics*. AAFP Reprint No. 279. http://www.aafp.org/dam/AAFP/documents/medical_education_residency/program_directors/Reprint279_Ethics.pdf. Accessed December 2, 2016.

45. Slowther A, Fulford B, Peile E, Dale J. *Clinical Ethics and Values-Based Practice: Curriculum Statement* 3.3. Royal College of General Practitioners. http://www.gmc-uk.org/3_3_Ethics_2006_

01.pdf_30448781.pdf. Published September 2005. Updated February 2007. Accessed November 19, 2016.

46. Royal College of General Practitioners. *Curriculum for Australian General Practice 2016 CS16 Core Skills Unit*. Royal Australian College of General Practitioners. http://www.racgp.org.au/education/curriculum/2016-curriculum/. Accessed November 19, 2016.

47. Pauls MA. Teaching and evaluation of ethics and professionalism in Canadian family medicine residency programmes. *Can Fam Physician*. 2012, 58: 751–756. https://www.ncbi.nlm.nih.gov/pubmed/23242906.

48. Manson H, Satin D, Nelson V, Vadiveloo T. Ethics education in family medicine training in the United States: A national survey. *Fam Med*. 2014, 46(1): 28–35. http://www.stfm.org/FamilyMedicine/Vol46Issue1/Manson28.

49. Schuh LA, Burdette DE. Initiation of an effective neurology resident ethics curriculum. *Neurology*. 2004; 62(10): 1897–1898. https://www.ncbi.nlm.nih.gov/pubmed/15159507.

50. Sulmasy DP, Marx ES. Ethics education for medical house officers: Long term improvements in knowledge and confidence. *J Med Ethics*. 1997; 23: 88–92. https://www.ncbi.nlm.nih.gov/pmc/articles/PMC1377207/.

51. Alfandre D, Rhodes R. Improving ethics education during residency training. *Med Teach*. 2009; 31: 513–517. https://www.ncbi.nlm.nih.gov/pubmed/19811167.

52. Levin A, Berry S, Kassarardjian C, Howard F, McKneally MF. Ethics teaching is as important as my clinical education: A survey of participants in residency at a single university. *UTMH*. 2006; 84(1): 60–63.

53. Manson H. The need for medical ethics education in family medicine training. *Fam Med*. 2008; 40(9): 658–664. http://www.stfm.org/FamilyMedicine/Vol46Issue1/Manson28.

54. Eilat-Tsanani S, Notzer N, Lavi I, Tabenkin H. Medical ethics: Training residents in family medicine. *Educ Prim Care*. 2008; 19: 303–312. http://www.tandfonline.com/doi/abs/10.1080/14739879.2008.11493686.

55. Daniels K. Integration of ethics teaching within GP training. *Educ Prim Care*. 2012; 23(2):75–78. PMID: 2244945.

56. Chamberlain J, Nisker J. Residents' attitudes to training in ethics in Canadian obstetrics and gynecology programmes. *Obstet*

Gyncol. 1995; 85(6): 783–786. http://www.sciencedirect.com/science/article/pii/002978449500019N.

57. Berseth C, Durand R. Evaluating the effect of a human values seminar on ethical attitudes toward resuscitation among pediatric residents. *Mayo Clin Proc.* 1990; 65(3): 337–343. https://www.ncbi.nlm.nih.gov/pubmed/2314123.

58. Sulmasy D, Geller G, Levine D, Faden R. A randomized trial of ethics education for medical house officers. *J Med Ethics.* 1993; 19(3): 157–163. PMCID: PMC1376284.

59. Wada K, Doering M, Rudnick A. Ethics education for psychiatry residents: A mixed-design retrospective evaluation of an introductory course and a quarterly seminar. *Camb Q Healthc Ethics.* 2013; 22(4): 425–435. https://doi.org/10.1017/S0963180113000339.

60. Bloch, S, Green, S.A. Promoting the teaching of psychiatric ethics. *Acad Psychiatry.* 2009; 33(2): 89–92. https://doi.org/10.1176/appi.ap.33.2.89.

61. Accreditation Council for Graduate Medical Education and American Board of Psychiatry and Neurology. *The Psychiatry Milestone Project.* https://www.acgme.org/Portals/0/PDFs/Milestones/PsychiatryMilestones.pdf. Published July 2015. Accessed December 7, 2016.

62. Royal College of Psychiatrists. *A Competency Based Curriculum for Specialist Core Training in Psychiatry.* http://www.rcpsych.ac.uk/pdf/CORE_CURRICULUM_2010_Mar_2012_update.pdf. Published February 2010. Updated March 2012. Accessed December 7, 2016.

63. Royal College of Physicians and Surgeons of Canada. *Objective of Training in the Specialty of Psychiatry.* http://www.royalcollege.ca/cs/groups/public/documents/document/mdaw/mdg4/~edisp/088003.pdf. Published July 15, 2015. Accessed November 29, 2016.

64. Coverdal JH, Bayer T, Isbell P, Moffic S. Are we teaching psychiatrists to be ethical? *Acad Psychiatry,* 1992; 16(4): 199–205. https://doi.org/10.1007/BF03341393.

65. Ping I, Guedet PJ. Ethics and professionalism preparation for psychiatrists-in-training: A curricular proposal. *Int Rev Psychiatry.* 2010; 22(3): 301–305. https://doi.org/10.3109/09540261.2010.482095.

66. Roberts LW, McCarty T, Roberts BB, Morrison N, Belitz J, Berenson C, Siegler M. Clinical ethics teaching in psychiatric supervision. *Acad Psychiatry.* 1996; 20(3): 176–188. https://doi.org/10.1007/BF03341568.

67. Roberts LW, McCarty T, Lyketsos C, Hardee JT, Jacobson J, Walker R, Siegler M. What and how psychiatry residents at ten training programmes wish to learn about ethics. *Acad Psychiatry.* 1996; 20(3): 131–143. https://doi.org/10.1007/BF03341563.

68. Gupta M, Forlini C, Lenton K, et al. A minimum standard of ethics? A qualitative study the hidden ethics curriculum in two Canadian psychiatry residency programmes. *Acad Psychiatry.* 2016; 40: 592. https://doi:10.1007/s40596-015-0456-0

69. Hoop JG. Hidden ethical dilemmas in psychiatric residency training: The psychiatry resident as dual agent. *Acad Psychiatry.* 2004; 28(3): 183–189. https://doi.org/10.1176/appi.ap.28.3.183.

70. *The Future of Medical Education—Postgraduate Project Report: A Collective Vision for Postgraduate Medical Education.* https://afmc.ca/future-of-medical-education-in-canada/postgraduate-project/phase2/index.php. Published 2012. Accessed December 7, 2016.

71. Dingle AD, Stuber ML. Ethics education. *Child Adolesc Psychiatr Clin N Amer.* 2008; 17(1): 187–207. https://doi.org/10.1016/j.chc.2007.07.009.

72. See also Rudin E, Edelson R, Servis M. Literature as an introduction to psychiatric ethics. *Acad Psychiatry.* 1998; 22(1): 41–46. https://doi.org/10.1007/BF03341443.

73. Wada K, Doering M, Rudnick A. Ethics education for psychiatry residents: A mixed-design retrospective evaluation of an introductory course and a quarterly seminar. *Camb Q Healthc Ethics.* 2013; 22(4): 425–435. https://doi.org/10.1017/S0963180113000339.

74. Green B, Miller PD, Routh CP. Teaching ethics in psychiatry: A one-day workshop for clinical students. *J Med Ethics.* 1995; 21(4): 234–238.

75. Keune JD, Kodner IJ. The importance of an ethics curriculum in surgical education. *World J Surg.* 2014; 38(7):1581–1586.

76. Howard F, McKneally, MF, Upshur RE, Levin AV. The formal and informal surgical ethics curriculum: Views of resident and staff surgeons in Toronto. *Am J Surg.* 2012; 203(2):358–365.

77. Helft PR, Eckles RE, Torbeck L. Ethics education in surgical residency programs: A review of the literature. *J Surg Educ.* 2009; 66(1): 35–42.

78. Downing MT, Way DP, Caniano DA. Results of a national survey on ethics education in general surgery residency programs. *Am J Surg.* 1997; 174(3): 364–368.

79. Royal College of Physicians and Surgeons of Canada. Bioethics. http://www.royalcollege.ca/rcsite/bioethics-e. Accessed January 9, 2017.

80. McAlister C. Breaking the silence of the switch—Increasing transparency about trainee participation in surgery. *N Engl J Med.* 2015; 372(6): 2477–2479. doi:10.1056/NEJMp1502091

81. Gawande A. The learning curve. *The New Yorker.* January 28, 2002. http://www.newyorker.com/magazine/2002/01/28/the-learning-curve. Accessed November 29, 2016.

82. The 6th Halifax Ethics Symposium in Ophthalmology 2015. https://medicine.dal.ca/content/dam/dalhousie/pdf/faculty/medicine/departments/department-sites/opthamology/Ethics%20Symposium%202015.pdf. Accessed November 29, 2016.

83. Dalrymple J, Abbott J, Buery-Joyner S, et al. Online objective teaching cases and outlines. Association of Professors of Gynecology and Obstetrics. https://www.apgo.org/component/content/article/ 31-objectives/329-online-objective-teaching-cases-and-outlines.html. Accessed November 19, 2016.

84. Royal College of Surgeons. Homepage. https://www.rcseng.ac.uk/. Accessed November 26, 2016.

85. American College of Surgeons. Ethical Issues in Clinical Surgery. https://www.facs.org/education/division-of-education/publications/ethicalissuesinclinicalsurgery. Accessed November 26, 2016.

86. Brewster LP, et al. Assessing residents in surgical ethics: We do it a lot; we only know a little. *J Surg Res.* 2011; 171(2):395–398.

87. Carrese J, McDonald E, Moon M, et al. Everyday ethics in internal medicine resident clinic: An opportunity to teach. *Med Educ.* 2011; 45(7): 711–725. doi:10.1111/j1365-2923.2011.03931.x

88. Daboval T, Ferretti E, Moore G. Innovative holistic teaching in a Canadian neonatal perinatal medicine residency program. *Hastings Cent Rep.* 2014; 44: 21–25. doi:10.1002/hast.384

89. Taylor H, McDonald E, Moon M, et al. Teaching ethics to pediatric residents: The centrality of the therapeutic alliance. *Med Educ.* 2009; 43(10): 952–959. doi:10.1111/j1365-2923.2009.03449.x

90. Royal College of Physicians and Surgeons of Canada. *Objectives of Training in Pediatrics.* http://www.royalcollege.ca/cs/groups/public/documents/document/y2vk/mdaw/~edisp/tztest3rcpsced000931.pdf. Published 2008. Accessed January 30, 2017.

91. Royal Australasian College of Physicians. Physician Readiness for Expert Practice (PREP) Training Program. General Paediatrics Advanced Training Curriculum. https://www.racp.edu.au/docs/default-source/default-document-library/at-general-paediatrics-curricula.pdf?sfvrsn=2. Published 2010. Updated 2013. Accessed January 30, 2017.

92. Accreditation Council for Graduate Medical Education and American Academy of Pediatrics. The Pediatrics Milestone Project. https://www.acgme.org/Portals/0/PDFs/Milestones/PediatricsMilestones.pdf. Published July 2007. Accessed January 30, 2017.

93. Wagner P, Hendrich J, Moseley G, Hudson V. Defining medical professionalism: A qualitative study. *Med Educ.* 2007; 41(3): 288–294.

94. Diekema DS, Shugerman RP. An ethics curriculum for the pediatric residency program confronting barriers to implementation. *Arch Pediatr Adolesc Med.* 1997; 151(6): 609–614.

95. Lang CW, Smith PJ, Ross LF. Ethics and professionalism in the pediatric curriculum: A survey of pediatric program directors. *Pediatrics.* 2009; 12(4): 1143–1151.

96. Cook AF, Sobotks SA, Ross LF. Teaching and assessment of ethics and professionalism: A survey of pediatric program directors. *Acad Pediatr.* 2013; 13(6): 570–576.

97. 1 Kesselheim JC, Najita J, Morley D, Bair E, Joffe S. Ethics knowledge of recent pediatric residency graduates: The role of residency ethics curricula. *J Med Ethics.* 2016, 4(2): 809–814.

98. Boyte WR. Casey's Legacy. *Health Affairs.* 2001; 20(2):250–254. doi:10.1377/hlthaff.20.2.250

99. Hilfiker D. Facing our mistakes. *N Engl J Med.* 1984; 310(2): 118–122. doi:10.1056/NEJM198401123100211

100. Kesselheim JC, Sectish TC, Joffe S. Education in professionalism: Results from a survey of pediatric residency program directors. *J Grad Med Educ.* 2012; 4(1): 101–105.

101. Rosenbluth G, O'Brien B, Asher EM, Cho CS. The "zing factor"—how do faculty describe the best pediatrics residents? *J Grad Med Educ*. 2014; 6(1): 106–111.

102. Warren AE, Allen VM, Bergin F, Hazelton L, Alexadis-Brown P, Lightfoot K, McSweeney J, Singleton J, Sargeant J, Mann K. Understanding, teaching and assessing the elements of the CanMEDS professional role: Canadian program directors' views. *Med Teach*. 2104, 36(5): 390–402. doi:10.3109/0142159X.2014.890281

103. What is ethics? *BBC*. http://www.bbc.co.uk/ethics/introduction/intro_1.shtml. Accessed April 16, 2017.

104. Stirrat GM. Reflections on learning and teaching medical ethics in UK medical schools. *J Med Ethics*. 2015; 41(1): 8–11.

105. College of Physicians and Surgeons of Ontario. http://www.cpso.on.ca/Policies-Publications/The-Practice-Guide-Medical-Professionalism-and-Col/Introduction

5

The Visible Curriculum

EVA-MARIE STERN AND SHELLEY WALL

The Hidden and the Visible

The hidden curriculum is an acknowledged part of medical training; it consists in "the commonly held 'understandings,' customs, rituals, and taken-for-granted aspects of what goes on in the life-space we call medical education."[1] Critics speak of the ways the hidden curriculum shapes learners' outlooks with a set of pungent biases, assumptions and prejudices.[2] These are instilled through the expressions, tones, and attitudes of their peers and role models, often without words, in the manner of an environmental or relational aesthetic[3] in which students are immersed, live, and learn. More outspoken scholars describe how paternalism and negligence[4] are among the values transmitted in this way; and wherever unacknowledged and tacit they reproduce transgenerationally,[5] resulting in damage to doctors' well-being as well as that of their patients.[6]

The *visible* curriculum—our term for the use of visual arts in medical education across all levels of training—has for several decades taken its place among other humanities offerings as a means to illuminate and address these ills. In published accounts of humanistic medical education the visual arts emerge alongside the "liberal arts" of history, literature, and philosophy as early as 1983.[7] Innovations in our times feature art as an agent for questioning and transforming perceptions of issues such as human rights, equity, identity, illness, treatment, and the process of healing.[8] In this chapter, we summarize current visual teaching/learning modalities used in medical training, consider the importance of art-*making* in addition to art observation, suggest differences in approach between undergraduate and residency training, and offer some practical examples of visual arts–based sessions for training and reflection.

Literature Review

Among humanities initiatives now widely undertaken by medical schools across Canada, the United States, and the United Kingdom, narrative medicine involving reflective writing and the reading of literary texts is the most common modality (see chapter 3); however, more recently, medical schools have begun to include visual methods in their health humanities offerings. These are more commonly implemented at the undergraduate level and are often offered as electives rather than core curriculum. In addition to arts-based curricula, numerous medical schools, including our own, have artist-in-residence programs, in which embedded artists work with medical trainees, staff, patients, and the wider community. It is not uncommon for medical schools to mount exhibitions of student and resident artwork. Such initiatives speak not only to the expansion of health humanities but to the increasing "dominance of the visual" in contemporary culture.[9]

A literature search was conducted using the Medline database to identify research related to the use of visual arts in medical education; following up on the reference lists of articles identified through this means yielded further results. Among 51 published reports of specific curricular initiatives incorporating the viewing or creation of visual art in medical training, 40 reported on undergraduate-level medical curricula that were visual arts–based or included visual art among other modalities, while only 11 reported on similar initiatives exclusively for, or involving, learners at the postgraduate/residency level. We include undergraduate initiatives in our review here, first to consider the insights these offer into the efficacy of visual methods in healthcare training generally and second as a basis for considering differences in the role of visual arts in undergraduate and postgraduate curricula. Where published reports on curricula for faculty development, interprofessional education, or students in nursing or allied health professions offer insights that may be useful to postgraduate medical education, we include those as well. In addition to the literature search, we supplemented our view of the field through phone interviews with key informants involved in visual arts–based health humanities programs at a number of North American medical schools.

Looking

The purposes of having medical trainees view artworks have been framed in various ways. These might be loosely grouped into four kinds of objective:

1. the sharpening of technical abilities, such as close observation, diagnostic acumen, pattern recognition, and the perception of nonverbal cues;[10-12]
2. the fostering of cognitive skills, such as description and interpretation (and understanding the distinction between them), critical thinking, and metacognition (critical awareness of the process of learning);[13-15]
3. the development of interpersonal skills with both patients and colleagues, such as communication, collaboration, social awareness, and cultural sensitivity;[16-19] and
4. personal growth: professional identity formation and the nurturing of humanistic qualities such as empathy, tolerance of ambiguity, creativity, and enhanced self-reflection.[20-24]

These objectives map to core competencies in medical education and to the roles residents are learning to inhabit, such as communicator, collaborator, advocate, professional. These are by no means discrete or mutually exclusive categories: rather, all of these objectives build together to foster visually literate, sensitive, and humane practitioners. In all cases, trainees "struggle in a nonclinical but fraught environment to interpret complex and potentially conflicting meanings."[22] In other words, they are "learning to see" in ways that are highly relevant to core clinical skills. Visual literacy is the culmination of learning to see and to make meaning from what is observed. Braverman, among others, asserts that visual literacy is "a skill that cannot be taught formally by lecture, but only by experiential learning."[25] In the following paragraphs, we survey the locations where medical trainees might engage with visual art, the types of artwork that have been used to spark reflection, and some methods for facilitating art engagement, followed by examples of successful seminars or courses from the literature.

Museum visits are among the most common visual arts–based initiatives; these include facilitated observation of artworks and various forms of response to the work, such as discussions, written reflections, or drawing exercises based on the artworks on display. (Having medical trainees make art is discussed later.) In some cases, participants visit artists' studios rather than galleries, permitting engagement with both the art and its maker; in one program, medical students visited "patient-artists" in a studio space housed within a psychiatric facility, resulting in greater understanding of individuals living with chronic mental illness.[26] Some medical schools and teaching hospitals are situated in major centers, in proximity to art museums with which it is possible to initiate partnerships; some universities house both medical schools and institutional art museums. It is even possible to make use of the art displayed in hospitals, with the added benefit of having trainees reflect on the aesthetics and meanings, for patients and families, of the hospital environment.[16] When physical visits to galleries/museums/studios are not possible (due to time, cost, or location), online image banks, digital museum collections, and specialized image repositories make it possible to incorporate an infinite variety of high-quality visual art into humanities teaching (see the appendix for a list of such resources). Another art form that offers rich possibilities for interpretation, discussion, and the exercise of visual literacy is comics, or "graphic medicine,"[27] which may be easily engaged with in a classroom setting. There is a growing body of work in this area: see appendix for resources and links to a sample excercise.

Exploration of formal qualities is relevant as a first step to developing interpretive skills in medical encounters such as psychiatric assessments, physical examinations, and the interpretation of diagnostic images such as radiographs (see Box 5.1).

Some reports indicate the precise nature of the visual art that students engage with; others refer more generally to paintings, photographs, sculptures, or other media. For some educators, it seems that the artwork is primarily a vehicle for the representation of events, persons, interactions, and so on (the *what*), while the *how* of the representation—specifics of artistic style, composition, formal properties—is a less important part of the discussion.[28] Other studies, on the other hand, leverage the aesthetic qualities of individual artworks to deepen and complicate the experience of looking.[14] Abstract works, for example, have no *what*, no figurative narrative that can divert conversation from the material work itself; instead, students must confront the cognitively perplexing but psychologically affecting nature of nonrepresentational marks and come to realize a more complex burden of interpretive work.[22] This may be understood as an analogous task to learning to synthesize the meanings of a patient's presentation, where the verbal content of the complaint and the manner or *style* of his or her physical appearance can seem either consonant or clashing. Ambiguous, polyvalent works of art can also furnish an opportunity for collaborative meaning-making. For example, Katz and Khoshbin describe a museum-based, multidisciplinary team-building session in which participants confront "an extremely complex work of modern art that defies interpretation" and must collaborate together to interpret the piece.[29]

BOX 5.1 Major Aesthetic Elements To Be Observed in Artwork, Whether Representational or Abstract, and Questions to Guide Close Observation

Color: What colors are present; which are absent? Are they intense or pale, blended together, overlapping or kept separate? Does any color dominate the whole?

Value (light/dark): Does the overall piece appear more light or dark? Are there shadows? What is the lightest or brightest point of the artwork; what is the darkest?

Symmetry, balance, use of space, composition: To what degree is the overall piece symmetrical? What do you notice about its scale or size? Are there blank or unfinished spaces or spaces that appear very full?

Texture, pattern, rhythm: How flat versus three-dimensional does the art appear? Are there repeated patterns of marks? Do the marks give an overall appearance of multiplicity or sameness, fullness or sparseness?

Form, contour: Are there precise contours or are the edges of shapes indistinct? Are the shapes more geometric or organic?

Line pressure, emphasis: Are the lines fine or thick, broken or continuous? Is there a mark that catches your eye? Do the lines seem quickly or slowly made? with energy or not?

Movement, perspective: Where is your eye drawn first? Where does it go next? How far or close do you feel relative to the action in the image?

Numerous models for facilitating encounters with art exist. For example, Visual Thinking Strategies (VTS)[30] is a well-documented model of "learning to look," which has been successfully used in programs with residents.[29, 31,32] Based on the work of cognitive psychologist Abigail Housen, VTS seeks to grow learners' visual literacy, critical thinking, and communication skills—all capacities which are transferable to content areas other than the study of visual arts. A structured set of steps, including a series of simple prompts, provides a practical framework for guiding learners through their encounter with an artwork, for deepening their reflection on what they believe they observe and why, for facilitating group discussion, and for probing for the narrative arc(s) in a given work (see Box 5.2).

This structured approach to the artwork, with an emphasis on articulating the reasons for a particular interpretation or response, activates and questions assumptions—shared or not within a group— and provokes reflection on how they shape understanding. A museum-based undergraduate medical elective at the University of Toronto (see link to website at the end of the chapter) uses VTS to engage explicitly with the sociocultural and historical contexts of art and encourages learners to reflect on different practices of looking across time and across cultures. VTS's most obvious application is to representational artwork where landscapes, figures, and objects can be recognized in relation to each other. But it also aids in approaching abstract work where aesthetic elements such as color, shape, line, texture, and composition affect viewers' responses. It is not difficult to see how growing learners' confidence to engage with more ambiguous, multilevel, abstract work may translate into increasing their confidence with the necessary uncertainty and ambiguity which underlie much medical looking and figuring, in spite of increasingly precise visual diagnostic tools.

Similarly, the "personal responses tour" (PRT) is another form of in-museum viewing, in which participants are provided with

---

BOX 5.2 Three Questions Used in Visual Thinking Strategies to Enable Critical Thinking with Images

1. What's going on in this picture?
2. What do you see that makes you say that?
3. What more can we find?

Yenawine P. 2013. *Visual Thinking Strategies: Using Art to Deepen Learning Across School Disciplines*. Cambridge: Harvard Education Press; 2013.

reflection prompts to invite an emotional response to works of art—for example, "focus on a memorable patient of the past year, and find a work of art that person would find meaningful or powerful."[33] Participants explore the gallery on their own, identify an artwork, spend a period of reflection with it, and then act as "tour guide" to that work. Prompts may be varied to suit specific learning objectives. For example, in the "Art of Analysis" program at the Ohio State University College of Medicine students engage with artworks in a way that mirrors the process of encountering and planning treatment for patients, following a rubric for approaching museum artwork which echoes the procedure for conducting a medical assessment: Observe, Describe, Interpret and Prove.[34] With the help of prompts such as "What does compassion/empathy look like?", "What does being a good teacher look like?", or "Find a work of art that does/does not immediately appeal to you," learners explore the collection, choose an artwork, observe it closely, and present and discuss their findings with the group.

The artworks chosen in an art museum will, of course, depend on the museum's collection and the preferences of individual learners. In trainee-initiated museum viewing—as in, for instance, the personal responses tour—any artwork, even the most unexpected, might suggest meaningful connections in response to a prompt. Facilitator-led VTS sessions might be said to place a greater demand on the facilitator to choose work that is most likely to elicit rich themes for discussion—but here, too, it is the very nature of visual art to point in multiple directions, and so almost any artwork might provoke rich and unexpected responses. This openness encourages trainees to bring their own unprimed interpretations and responses into the learning space.

The original art accessible to learners will be different for each institution; almost any kind of art image may be found in reproduction; and the associations and interpretations stimulated by a work of art are likewise vast, depending on the learner, the facilitator, the collaborative meaning-making of a group, and the learning objectives of a course or seminar. For these reasons, rather than presenting a list of suggested artworks or prompts, we have chosen to provide illustrative examples of exercises in "looking." Table 5.1

TABLE 5.1 Selected Descriptions of Published Curricular Initiatives Using Visual Art

Facilitated or Self-Guided Encounter	Examples and Brief Descriptions	Objectives
Facilitated	The mandatory Brigham and Women's Hospital Internal Medicine Residency Humanistic Curriculum includes a "Night at the Museum of Fine Arts" structured on the VTS model. An initial exercise introduces VTS as a way to arrive at multiple interpretations of an object; subsequent exercises centered on preselected or trainee-chosen works encourage metaphorical thinking, connection-building, and reflections on themes such as professional identity, professional joys or struggles, and care for the dying. The night concludes with a relaxation meditation exercise in the museum's replica Buddhist temple.[29]	Foster resident well-being and humanistic qualities; prevent trainee burnout
	In the Mentored Writing course at Johns Hopkins University School of Medicine, each first-year psychiatry resident learns to distinguish observing from interpreting; reflect on and discuss their findings with others; present a poster; and complete a publication-ready essay about the human condition and its relevance to mental health, as evoked through an encounter with original artwork of their choice. Faculty time, two visits to art museums, the VTS framework, and *JAMA Psychiatry's* online Art and Images in Psychiatry collection comprise the resources for the five-day rotation. (One of the authors is developing an online version of the course for those who do not have access to museums.)[32]	Hone observational skills; learn about academic writing and manuscript submission; develop participants' perspectives on the human condition and on patients' experience of mental health; build group cohesion and morale

(continued)

TABLE 5.1 Continued

Facilitated or Self-Guided Encounter	Examples and Brief Descriptions	Objectives
	Introduction to the Clerkship Experience at Robert Wood Johnson Medical School includes an exercise that incorporates VTS into an expanded framework, using guided questions in viewing preselected artwork to elicit discussion related to Observation (O), Interpretation (I), Reflection (R), and Communication (C). The facilitator uses VTS questions to elicit descriptions of visual findings (O); learners are then invited to propose conclusions about the meaning of the artwork (I), to evaluate and question their conclusions (R), and to share their ideas (C).[15]	Train pre-clerkship students in observational skills necessary for clinical diagnosis
	The Art of Seeing program at McMaster University brings together residents from Family Medicine and ob/gyn and incorporates mindfulness, visual art, and dance within an art museum space. Each session builds upon the previous one: participants move from learning and applying the formal elements of art analysis (e.g., color, line, texture, movement), to examining the use of symbols as a means of visual communication, to encountering the ambiguities and challenges of contemporary and conceptual art. Participants create their own art and engage in reflective writing throughout the program. A session on dance reinforces an embodied understanding of the patient experience.[35]	Nurturing empathic, compassionate, and mindful behavior in residents

| Self-guided | The Personal Responses Tour has been used in a museum setting with groups of both undergraduate medical students and residents at Harvard Medical School. Participants are randomly assigned a reflection question to guide their selection of a work of art. Prompts include: "Find an image of a person with whom you find it difficult to empathize, and think about the barriers"; "Find a work of art from a culture or religious tradition other than your own, and identify something you find beautiful about the work"; "Find an object that for you expresses pure joy." Prompts can be crafted to suit any theme of interest. Each participant then leads a "tour" of the work they have chosen; the sharing of responses and group discussion is an important part of the intervention.[33] | Promote reflection, foster empathy, increase appreciation for the psychosocial context of patient experience, and create a space for learners to deepen relationships with one another |
| | The Personal Responses Tour (PRT) has been adapted to a hospital setting within the context of a mandatory Year 2 undergraduate medical education course at the National Taiwan University College of Medicine. This example of PRT is noteworthy on two counts: (a) it tests the transferability of PRT between cultures with different attitudes toward sharing thoughts and feelings and (b) in the absence of easy museum access, learners interacted with hospital artwork; this expediency had the added benefit of heightening trainees' awareness of the effects of the hospital environment on patients. The prompt used was "Choose a piece of art in the hospital that you would share with a sick child and explain why."[16] | Stimulate reflecting on empathy; sharing of reflections among medical trainees; community building |

(continued)

TABLE 5.1 Continued

Facilitated or Self-Guided Encounter	Examples and Brief Descriptions	Objectives
	In a pilot program at the Wellcome Museum (London), foundation trainees were invited to find a work of art which resonated with a clinical encounter or experience, to discuss it, and to articulate their response in a piece of writing structured according to a series of questions, moving from description to reflection. Themes in trainees' writing "concerned attitudes and assumptions about disease, understanding how their views and beliefs as doctors may be shaped by their world-view and appreciation of the nature of evidence-based practice."23	Reflection on clinical experiences; learning to see the familiar in unfamiliar ways

Note: VTS = Visual Thinking Strategies.

presents a partial selection of visual art-based curricula from the published literature. These examples are divided into encounters in which a facilitator pre-selects some of the artwork, and those in which learners are invited to make their own prompted choices within the museum space. Our curation of these examples has been made with a view to presenting curricula with a clearly defined, replicable structure (e.g., VTS, PRT). Table 5.2, on the other hand, takes its point of departure in the art itself; in it, we model the kinds of questions one might ask in viewing a given work of art and the kinds of imagery a facilitator might choose in order to get at particular themes or learning objectives. These examples

---

TABLE 5.2 Examples of the Kinds of Imagery a Facilitator Might Choose to Bring Out Particular Themes or Learning Objectives and Models of the Kinds of Questions to Ask

---

1. Susan Low-Beer: "Echos: Reflections on Structure," 2009. Board: mixed media and encaustic; koso paper: mixed media, board: approximately 30 x 21.5 in.; paper: 29 x 21.5 in. View online: http://susanlow-beer.com/echos-reflection/

From the artist's description: "This body of work consists of eight pieces. Each work has a pair. The two paintings are placed side by side [...]. The one is on a rigid board that projects from the wall two inches and is heavily painted with encaustic that continues around the sides. Its companion, translucent and surrounded by air, is painted on handmade Japanese paper in watercolour. It is attached to metal poles that come out from the wall two inches." (http://susanlow-beer.com/echos-reflection/)

Sample prompts to sharpen observational skills: What do you notice about the overall composition? its size? about the colors? about the shapes? Are the strokes heavy or light? Are the shapes/lines clear or obscure? Do they touch, overlap, or are they separate? Do the marks appear to have been made quickly or slowly? Do they go to the edges or not? Are they outlined or not? Does there appear to be movement in the images? Do they seem two- or three-dimensional? What are the similarities and differences between the two panels?

(continued)

TABLE 5.2 Continued

Sample prompts to invite interpretation and reflection: There are multiple, overlapping shapes in these images: what do you think is the most important shape and why? What is the least important and why? Do these panels remind you of places/of medical conditions/of forms of medical imagery? in what way? What do the material differences between these two panels suggest about their relationship? Does this relationship remind you of anything you have encountered in your clinical experience?

Objectives/themes addressed:
Pattern recognition; tolerating and deciphering ambiguity; appreciating multiple interpretations of a phenomenon

2. Rebecca Belmore: "Fringe," 2007. Photograph in light box, 96 1/4 x 32 3/4 x 6 1/2 in. National Gallery of Canada.
View online: https://humanrights.ca/sites/default/files/Belmore_Fringe_Media_02.jpg

Details: the gash was created with special-effects makeup, and the blood is made of beads

Sample prompts to sharpen observational skills: What do you notice about the size and orientation of this photograph? What do you notice about the figure depicted? about how he/she is arranged in the frame of the picture? how close or far he/she is from the viewer? about the marks on his/her skin? how he/she is clothed? about the color and texture of his/her skin? What do you notice about the quality of the sutures? What is shown in addition to the figure? What are the dominant colors/shapes? What do you notice about the lighting?

Sample prompts to invite interpretation and reflection: How does viewing this artwork make you feel? What do you think happened to the person depicted? What is your relationship as viewer to the person depicted here? What do you not see? Does it make a difference to know that the artist is a woman? What, if anything, can we know for certain about the gender, race, or age of this figure? When do you think this work was made and why? Does it affect your interpretation to know that the Anishinaabe artist who created this photograph is known for using her work to address the history of violence and oppression against indigenous peoples?

TABLE 5.2 Continued

Objectives/themes addressed:
Embodiment; the medical gaze; cultural perspectives on health; history of medicine; empathy

3. Christi Belcourt: "Water Song," c. 2014. Acrylic on canvas, approximately 12 x 7.5 feet. National Gallery of Canada.
View online: http://christibelcourt.com/ancestry/ngc72dpi16in/

Description: Belcourt replicates the look of traditional Métis beadwork by building up images out of tiny dots of acrylic paint.

Prompts to sharpen observational skills: What do you notice about the size of this work? What do you notice about the overall composition? about the pattern of the elements within it? Do the elements touch, overlap, or are they separate? Where are the lines finest? What colors dominate? Where is the work symmetrical? Where is it asymmetrical? How are the individual marks made?

Prompts to invite interpretation and reflection: What is the relationship of the parts to the whole? of foreground to background? What does this painting say about health? about bodies? about nature? about relationships? If this was an image of a bodily organ, which organ would it be and why? Could this be an x-ray, a CT scan, or an MRI and why? What is the significance of plants in medicine, historically and in contemporary practices?

Objectives/themes addressed:
Pattern recognition; interpretation of symbols; embodiment; interdependency; cultural perspectives on health

are by no means prescriptive: they are meant to illustrate possible approaches to looking. It is our hope that these examples will stimulate educators' own creativity in developing visual curricula.

Making

Initiatives in the realm of "having medical students make stuff"[36] are less common than those that have trainees engage through observation, but in the past few years art-making arises increasingly in the reports of health-humanities educators.[8,37,38]

Exercises in *visual* art-making specifically range from the instrumental to the purely reflective. On the instrumental side, for example, medical trainees may learn and practice the basics of graphical language to equip them to use sketching as a means of communication with patients and colleagues[39] or to consolidate anatomical knowledge.[40] At the reflective end of the spectrum, medical trainees are encouraged to use art-making (specifically visual art, or visual art as an option among other modalities) to express and process their thoughts and feelings and to reflect on clinical experiences.[17,20,34,41–50] Art-making (e.g., painting, drawing, collage, photography) may happen as part of a facilitated session or be assigned as a reflective exercise to be completed on the trainee's own time. It is also possible to have medical trainees participate alongside patients in art-making exercises,[51] as in the "shadowing artists on the wards" elective in Edmonton, Alberta, in which medical students are paired with artists-in-residence working at the bedside.[52] Such exercises not only provide trainees with a creative outlet for their own experience but provide them with first-hand insight into the patient experience. Yet another kind of art-making happens at Penn State College of Medicine, where fourth-year medical students have been working within the context of a seminar series to create comics reflective of their professional identity formation; this exercise has been shown to enhance a host of competencies, from clinical reasoning skills to empathy.[20] It is also possible to use art-making by medical trainees as a diagnostic tool in itself: in a study by Julliard and colleagues, for example, the analytical techniques of art therapy were used to analyze drawings made by family practice residents for themes related to stress.[53] Kelly and colleagues note the potential of trainee artwork "as a tool to evaluate student learning in medical education."[43]

Life-drawing (drawing from a nude model) occupies a pivotal place at the intersection between clinical and humanistic ways of looking and between instrumental goals (consolidating observational skills) and reflective, empathic ones (experiencing an embodied encounter with another person). Some museum-based programs incorporate life drawing as part of the experience.[14,29,54] At the University of Toronto, the "Looking Through Art" elective pairs museum visits with life-drawing sessions led by an artist as a way to provide "complementary but unique methods for students to explore the roles of looking, touch and representation in medical practice."[55] An innovative program at the University of Brighton pairs medical students with students in a three-dimensional design (craft) degree; these teams engage in collaborative drawing foregrounding the human body and in the process benefit from the exchange of perspectives from radically different disciplines. This program's emphasis on the human body as subject highlights "the nature of drawing as a deeply physical, sensory experience."[19] As drawing researcher Lucy Lyons puts it, in observational drawing we *participate with* what we are observing; we spend time noticing and in doing so invest the object of our drawing with dignity. Drawing is "a phenomenological activity that initiates and engenders knowledge."[56] Lyons' reference to dignity suggests a further benefit of art-making: artistic creation born out of slow, deliberate noticing and attention to the feel of materials involves *taking care*, in both observation and action.

In all such art-making, "creativity" emerges as a crucial quality in clinical training: the ability to respond to problematic or ambiguous situations with flexibility and innovation.[37] Creative work by its very nature requires innovative approaches to problem-solving and offers a "safe space" to fail[36] or, put another way, cultivates "comfort in not-knowing."[37] Gaufberg and Williams refer to the state of "beginner's mind"—a concept from Zen Buddhism now often invoked in mindfulness training—encouraged in residents as they view art in a museum;[33] this state of fresh seeing is even more heightened when a learner is actually engaged in creation.

Residency and Embodiment

"At its best, the learning of residents is participatory, developmental and progressive, and situated and distributed."[57]

Whereas medical school is tasked with providing a heft of theo-retical knowledge, in residency students become progressively immersed and responsible for acting on their understanding, for moving "ultimately beyond discussions to action in the world."[58]

This developmental continuum, from learning to see to learning to engage, finds an analogue in the spectrum of visual arts methods offered throughout medical education. Where under-graduate medical education teaches how to navigate the map, post-graduate medical education places doctors more and more firmly as agents on the terrain. But both undergraduate and graduate med-ical education provide a zigzag course between theory and practice, creating a "blurred edge,"[59] rather than a distinct line between the two. Specialty training, however, requires a deeper involvement with patients. Similarly, art-related exercises of both the looking and the making varieties are offered at both levels, but the mes-sier process of *making* mirrors the greater personal/professional invitations and demands of residency.

Making visual art—whether it be drawing, painting, collage, sculpture, or some other incarnation—engages not only the eyes and mind but the body. It involves physical interaction with the material world: an embodied practice. Some arts-based training initiatives explicitly integrate visual art-making with other embodied forms of art, such as dance.[35,54] (Other examples of exercises encouraging embodied practice/presence can be found in chapter 7.) Art histo-rian James Elkins suggests that, in looking at pictures of the body, "the pictured body is no longer imagined as an immobile shape on paper or canvas, but as a counterpart and figure for the observer."[60] This somatic empathy with other bodies is even more germane when the viewer is also a maker, tracing the vectors of an observed body, as in figure drawing, or working nonrepresentationally with the tactile materials of art.

"We looked at artists' painted self-portraits and later we made some scribbles and some clay pieces. [. . .] I don't know what happened—I didn't know that sometimes not even knowing what I was looking at, and then not knowing how [to] use clay, could help me *get it*—get it about bodies, and skin, and people, and about myself."[61]

Art-making activates skills essential to medical care which go beyond words and beyond cognitive work. A process as simple as making marks on paper or representing pain with a lump of clay[62] offers a medium for synthesizing and embodying understanding. "[B]ecause it may tap into unconscious, tacit beliefs and insights in ways that otherwise may not be easily accessible,"[58] original artwork may help surface learners' struggles with the hidden curriculum and their own unword-able but essential experiential growth, so that struggles and growth may be witnessed and understood by learners themselves, their peers, and their educators.[8] (See link to website at the end of the chapter for an example of group art-making which addresses approaches to the doctor-patient relationship in this way.) Visual narratives (explicit or implied in painting, drawing, sculpture) "represent another, and often invisible, component of the illness experience because they are 'right-brain' nonlinear depictions of the tacit, intuitive, emotional, and holistic nuances generally referred to as the 'aesthetic experience.'"[41]

Incorporating Visual Arts–Based Methods into Residency Training: Challenges and Recommendations

All the residents, doctors, and educators involved in arts-based education interviewed for this chapter agreed on the need for the visual arts to be embedded officially in clinical learning, rather than as (interesting but) extraneous activities. It is currently unusual for visual arts–based programs to form part of the core curriculum within undergraduate medical education (for an example of integrating visual studies throughout themes such as anatomy, cadaver study, life cycles, and professional identity, see Boisaubin and Winkler[63]) and even more rare for it to be a mandatory component in residency training. Many authors note the difficulty of finding time in an already full curriculum, especially for the arts.[23,36] Other barriers include funding, personnel, and institutional support. Many of the challenges involved in integrating visual arts into residency training are common to other medical humanities initiatives and are addressed elsewhere in this volume; what follow are some observations on curricular integration and faculty development as they relate specifically to visual arts–based methods.

Curricular Integration

Shapiro and Rucker articulate the critical concepts of "horizontal coherence" and "vertical complexity" in designing longitudinal arts-based programs. Where "horizontal coherence" describes the integration of humanities programs with concurrent clinical or course-work, "vertical complexity" describes the way in which a longitudinal program "progressively introduces concepts and methods of greater depth and intricacy"[64]—for example, by moving from the cognitive domain of visual literacy to the more humanistic values crucial to whole-patient care. This distinction is succinctly illustrated in Katz and Khoshbin's description, within a single article, of museum-based programs using VTS for, on the one hand, first-year medical students and, on the other, first-year residents. In the first instance, an elective combining museum visits and lectures applied the skills of close observation, description, analysis, communication, and collaboration exercised in the museum to the practice of competencies in physical diagnosis. In the second instance, residents were guided to engage with artworks in ways that connected them to humanistic values, with the objective of promoting resident well-being and preventing burnout.[29]

Indeed, the focus on physician well-being by way of arts-based practices comes to the fore in reports of residency-level programs. Self-reflection was a recurrent theme in descriptions of visual arts interventions for residents. Of the 11 articles on residency-based arts programs identified in our literature review, six of them included and even prioritized self-care, the alleviation and/or exploration of physicians' emotional engagement, stress, and risk of burnout or "dehumanization."[29,32,33,35,41,53] Engagement with art within a rotation provides a space for sanctioned "play" away from the high-stakes stress of clinical work; at the same time, it provides an opportunity for potentially transformative meditation on, and sharing of responses to, those clinical encounters.

Faculty and Facilitation

Medical schools with the most well-developed arts curricula count faculty with backgrounds in the visual arts, in addition to their medical or educational training. It may be that these departments in turn attract faculty who implement teaching via their creative medium. Medical visual humanities educators are devoted to their cause; programs that propose the arts are most often created and sustained by individuals who innovate rather than deliver prepackaged or traditional curricula. Having a supervisor or mentor versed in the arts may model creative, outside-the-box thinking as well as a comfort with uncertainty.[37] For this reason, succession planning in the visual humanities can be a barrier to the longevity of programs. It is important, as noted by Shapiro and Rucker, to build faculty development into arts-based programs[64] so that faculty who may not have a humanities background will be both inspired and equipped to facilitate future sessions. This may be accomplished, for example, by having faculty members who are not yet involved in teaching humanities attend arts-based sessions, to familiarize themselves with the curriculum and with discipline-specific approaches and as a form of mentoring.[65]

Ideally, gallery and museum visits and art-making endeavors are co-facilitated by educators from the medical, artistic, and curatorial sides. Where specific artistic practices, such as life-drawing, are included, it is essential to pair with an artist and/or arts educator. Not only in the scope of making but in the pursuit of learning to look actively as well, visual artists offer crucial guidance. "There is a vital aesthetic dimension to clinical judgement,"[66] and as such the artist's sensibility teaches learners to see beyond preconceived signs, to notice fresh visual phenomena. Bleakley in particular argues for the input of the artist in training the clinician's eye and mind.[66] Such partnerships may require funding to pay artists and educators from outside the medical school, or they may be accomplished through collaboration with faculty from other departments within an institution.

In using artwork for educational ends and choosing pieces to fit a target theme, educators risk flattening rich, storied, nuanced, and beautiful work into mere illustrations of ideas. This instrumental use of art is akin to approaching patients as examples of course material rather than apprehending each as a person with a singular context and history. As Boisaubin and Winkler note, an antidote comes in the form of the artist's expertise in helping learners identify the formal elements of a work[63]—a kind of care-full "aesthetic labor"[4]—and to appreciate the ways these shape its meaning. A doctor who understands how form coalesces with substance[67] is well prepared to see his or her patients as a creation of their own time, place, race, position, life experience, and relationships.

Conclusion

The experience of medical school is, among other things, a process of enculturation. In the modern era, Foucault would have us see the doctor-in-training as learning to use his or her gaze as an instrument of dissection—excising the patient's self from his or her body—to better divide and conquer illness.[68] Humanities scholars have refocused the learner's lens on understanding and learning to treat the patient as a whole person and, as a necessary correlate, learning to attend to his or her own personal/professional needs. To do so, the field of health humanities is calling for the doctor's aperture to open wide enough to consider his or her whole self as the instrument of healing. Since the inception of health humanities, medical educators have asked learners to refine not only their observational skills but also their social and emotional intelligence. This evolution has allowed a crucial shift: from learning the medical gaze, to engaging in clinical service: from *looking* to *making*.

Traditional medical training presents an anaesthetic picture.[4] The qualities of the science-based curriculum may be compared to the tenets of modernism: abstraction (and paradoxically, literalness), collage, minimalism, functionalism, and futurism.[69] These traits reflect and promote fragmentation and de-contextualization. "Without a humanist perspective, a patient might easily be represented—and treated—atomistically, as no more than a collection of organs and systems."[70] In contrast, movements in art such as the Renaissance posit as essential an awareness of context and one's participation in the scene, perspective, as well as a grounding in place, time, and social structures. Similarly, a humanities-strong learning environment calls for an infusion of embodied practice.

Parallel to the art/historic evolution, we can consider the continuum of teachings, from the beginning of medical school to the end of residency, as a progression from learning the modernist sensibilities of vocabulary, anatomy, physiology, taxonomies, and classifications; through integrating concepts into practice; into a renewed apprehension of one's patient as an other[71,72] by involving one's whole self in the healing relationship.

A sample curriculum to accompany this chapter can be found online at http://cahh.ca/resources/ouplesson-plans/.

References

1. Hafferty FW. Beyond curriculum reform: confronting medicine's hidden curriculum. *Acad Med.* 1998; 73:403–407.
2. Gupta M, Forlini C, Lenton K, Duchen R, Lohfeld L. The hidden ethics curriculum in two Canadian psychiatry residency programs: a qualitative study. *Acad Psychiatr.* 2016; 40(4):592–599.

3. Bollas C. *The Shadow of the Object: Psychoanalysis of the Unthought Known*. London: Free Association Books; 1987.

4. Bleakley A. The medical humanities in medical education: toward a medical aesthetics of resistance. In: Jones T, Wear D, Friedman LD, eds., *Health Humanities Reader*. New Brunswick, NJ: Rutgers University Press; 2014.

5. Michalec B, Hafferty FW. Stunting professionalism: the potency and durability of the hidden curriculum within medical education. *Soc Theor Health*. 2013; 11(4):388–406.

6. Bleakley A, Marshall R. Can the science of communication inform the art of the medical humanities? *Med Educ*. 2013; 47(2):126–133.

7. Berg G, ed. *The Visual Arts and Medical Education*. Carbondale and Edwardsville: Southern Illinois University Press; 1983.

8. Kumagai AK. Acts of interpretation: a philosophical approach to using creative arts in medical education. *Acad Med*. 2012; 87:1138–1144.

9. Metros SE. The educator's role in preparing visually literate learners. *Theor Pract*. 2008; 47(2):102–109.

10. Dolev JC, Friedlaender LK, Braverman IM. Use of fine art to enhance visual diagnostic skills. *JAMA*. 2001; 286:1020.

11. Friedlaender GE, Friedlaender LK. Art in science: enhancing observational skills. *Clin Orthop Relat R*. 2013; 471:2065–2067.

12. Shapiro J, Rucker L, Beck J. Training the clinical eye and mind: using the arts to develop medical students' observational and pattern recognition skills. *Med Educ*. 2006; 40(3):263–268.

13. Elder NC, Tobias B, Lucero-Criswell A, Goldenhar L. The art of observation: impact of a family medicine and art museum partnership on student education. *Fam Med*. 2006; 38(6):393–398.

14. Naghshineh S, Hafler JP, Miller AR, et al. Formal art observation training improves medical students' visual diagnostic skills. *J Gen Intern Med*. 2008; 23(7):991–997.

15. Jasani SK, Saks NS. Utilizing visual art to enhance the clinical observation skills of medical students. *Med Teach*. 2013; 35(7):e1327–e1331.

16. Ting S-W, Chen Y-Y, Ho M-J, Gaufberg E. Using hospital art in medical student reflection. *Med Educ*. 2012; 46:505–506.

17. Jones EK, Kittendorf AL, Kumagai AK. Creative art and medical student development: a qualitative study. *Med Educ*. 2017; 51:174–183.

18. Mininberg DT, Thompson N, Gillers D, Fins JJ. Commentary. *Acad Med*. 2004; 79(6):579.

19. Lyon P, Letschka P, Ainsworth T, Haq I. An exploratory study of the potential learning benefits for medical students in collaborative drawing: creativity, reflection and "critical looking." *BMC Med Educ*. 2013; 13(1):86.

20. Green MJ. Comics and medicine: peering into the process of professional identity formation. *Acad Med*. 2015; 90:774–779.

21. Zazulak J, Halgren C, Tan M, Grierson LEM. The impact of an arts-based programme on the affective and cognitive components of empathic development. *Med Humanit*. 2015; 41:69–74.

22. Schaff PB, Isken S, Tager RM. From contemporary art to core clinical skills: observation, interpretation, and meaning-making in a complex environment. *Acad Med*. 2011; 86:1272–1276.

23. Thresher K, Boreham L, Dennison L, Fletcher P, Owen C, Smith L, Scallan S. Exploring art with foundation doctors: reflecting on clinical experience. *Educ Prim Care*. 2013; 24(3):212–215.

24. Frich JC, Fugelli P. Medicine and the arts in the undergraduate medical curriculum at the University of Oslo Faculty of Medicine, Oslo, Norway. *Acad Med*. 2003; 78(10):1036–1038.

25. Braverman IM. To see or not to see: how visual training can improve observational skills. *Clin Dermatol*. 2011; 29(3):343–346.

26. Cutler JL, Harding KJ, Hutner LA, Cortland C, Graham MJ. Reducing medical students' stigmatization of people with chronic mental illness: a field intervention at the "living museum" State Hospital art studio. *Acad Psychiatr*. 2012; 36(3):191–196.

27. Czerwiec MK, Williams I, Squier SM, Green MJ, Myers KR, Smith ST. *The Graphic Medicine Manifesto*. University Park: Pennsylvania State University Press; 2015.

28. Bardes CL, Gillers D, Herman AE. Learning to look: developing clinical observational skills at an art museum. *Med Educ*. 2001; 35(12):1157–1161.

29. Katz JT, Khoshbin S. Can visual arts training improve physician performance? *Trans Am Clin Climatol Assoc*. 2014; 125(3):331–342.

30. Yenawine P. 2013. *Visual Thinking Strategies: Using Art to Deepen Learning Across School Disciplines*. Cambridge: Harvard Education Press; 2013.

31. Reilly JM, Ring J, Duke L. Visual thinking strategies: a new role for art in medical education. *Fam Med*. 2005; 37(4):250–252.

32. Leonpacher AK, Chisolm MS. Mentored writing: an arts-based curriculum for first-year psychiatry residents. *Acad Psychiatr.* 2016; 40:947–949.

33. Gaufberg E, Williams R. Reflection in a museum setting: the personal responses tour. *J Grad Med Educ.* 2011; 3:546–549.

34. Jacques A, Trinkley R, Stone L, Tang R, Hudson WWA, Khandelwal S. Art of analysis: a cooperative program between a museum and medicine. *J Learn Arts.* 2012; 8(1):1–10.

35. Zazulak J, Sanaee M, Frolic A, Knibb N, Tesluk E, Hughes E, Grierson LEM. The art of medicine: arts-based training in observation and mindfulness for fostering the empathic response in medical residents. *Med Humanit.* 2017; 43(3):192–198.

36. Green MJ, Myers K, Watson K, Czerwiec MK, Shapiro D, Draus S. Creativity in medical education: the value of having medical students make stuff. *Med Humanit.* 2016; 37:475–483.

37. Baruch JM, Jay M. Doctors as makers. *Acad Med.* 2016; 92(1):40–44.

38. Cox SM, Brett-Maclean P, Courneya CA. "My turbinado sugar": art-making, well-being and professional identity in medical education. *Arts Health.* 2016; 8:65–81.

39. Liou KT, George P, Baruch JM, Luks FI, Kevin T. Clinical sketches: teaching medical illustration to medical students. *Med Educ.* 2014; 48(5):525.

40. Bell LTO, Evans DJR. Art, anatomy, and medicine: Is there a place for art in medical education? *Anat Sci Educ.* 2014; 7:370–378.

41. Arnold BL, Lloyd LS, Von Gunten CF. Physicians' reflections on death and dying on completion of a palliative medicine fellowship. *J Pain Symptom Manag.* 2016; 5:633–639.

42. Graham J, Benson LM, Swanson J, Potyk D, Daratha K, Roberts K. Medical humanities coursework is associated with greater measured empathy in medical students. *Am J Med.* 2016; 129:1334–1337.

43. Kelly M, Bennett D, O'Flynn S. A picture tells 1000 words: learning teamwork in primary care. *Clin Teach.* 2013; 10(2):113–117.

44. LoFaso VM, Breckman R, Capello CF, Demopoulos B, Adelman RD. Combining the creative arts and the house call to teach medical students about chronic illness care. *J Am Geriatr Soc.* 2010; 58(2):346–351.

45. Magwood B, Casiro O, Hennen B. The medical humanities program at the University of Manitoba, Winnipeg, Manitoba, Canada. *Acad Med.* 2003; 78:1015–1019.
46. McBain L, Donnelly S, Hilder J, O'Leary C, McKinlay E. "I wanted to communicate my feelings freely": A descriptive study of creative responses to enhance reflection in palliative medicine education. *BMC Med Educ.* 2015; 15:180.
47. Rabow MW. Drawing on experience: physician artwork in a course on professional development. *Med Educ.* 2003; 37:1040–1041.
48. Shannon MT. Commentary [How do we communicate our experiences of daily life?]. *Acad Med.* 2013; 88(7):959.
49. Thompson T, Lamont-Robinson C, Younie L. "Compulsory creativity": rationales, recipes, and results in the placement of mandatory creative endeavour in a medical undergraduate curriculum. *Med Educ Online.* 2010; 15:1–8.
50. Weller K. Visualising the body in art and medicine: a visual art course for medical students at King's College Hospital in 1999. *Complement Ther Nurs Midwifery.* 2002; 8(2):211–216.
51. Roberts H, Noble J. Education research: changing medical student perceptions of dementia. *Neurology.* 2015; 85(8):739–741.
52. Brett-MacLean P, Casavant M, Serviss S, Cruz A. Shadowing artists on the wards: an undergraduate, arts-based medical elective. *Hektoen Int.* 2012; 4(1).
53. Julliard K, Intilli N, Ryan J, Vollmann S, Seshadri M. Stress in family practice residents: an exploratory study using art. *Art Ther.* 2002; 19(1):4–11.
54. De la Croix A, Rose C, Wildig E, Willson S. Arts-based learning in medical education: the students' perspective. *Med Educ.* 2011; 45(11):1090–100.
55. Crawford A. Personal correspondence with SW. June 11, 2017.
56. Lyons L. Drawing your way into understanding. *Tracey: Drawing and Visualisation Research.* May 2012. http://www.academia.edu/1598860/Drawing_your_way_into_understanding
57. Cooke M, Irby DM, O'Brien BC. *Educating Physicians: A Call for Reform of Medical School and Residency.* San Francisco, CA: Jossey-Bass; 2010.
58. Kumagai AK. From competencies to human interests. *Acad Med.* 2014; 89(7):978–983.
59. Stewart W. Interview with EMS. January 16, 2017.

60. Elkins J. *Pictures of the Body: Pain and Metamorphosis*. Stanford, CA: Stanford University Press; 1999.
61. Resident's seminar feedback [anonymous]. Telling Trauma Through Art course, University of Toronto; 2015.
62. Defenbaugh N. Interview with EMS. November 29, 2016.
63. Boisaubin E, Winkler M. Seeing patients and life contexts: the visual arts in medical education. *Am J Med Sci*. 2000; 319(5):292–296.
64. Shapiro J, Rucker L. Can poetry make better doctors? Teaching the humanities and arts to medical students and residents at the University of California, Irvine, College of Medicine. *Acad Med*. 2003; 78 953–957.
65. Zazulak J. Interview with SW. January 23, 2017.
66. Bleakley A, Farrow R, Gould D, Marshall R. Making sense of clinical reasoning: judgement and the evidence of the senses. *Med Educ*. 2003; 37:544–552.
67. Dewey J. *Art as Experience*. New York: Minton; 1934.
68. Foucault, Michel. *The Birth of the Clinic: An Archaeology of Medical Perception*, trans Sheridan AM. London and New York: Routledge; 2012.
69. McGilchrist I. *The Master and His Emissary: The Divided Brain and the Making of the Western World*. New Haven and London: Yale University Press; 2009.
70. Kidd MG, Connor JTH. Striving to do good things: teaching humanities in Canadian medical schools. *J Med Humanit*. 2008; 29(1):45–54.
71. Lévinas E. *Humanism of the Other*, trans. Poller N. Chicago: University of Illinois Press; 2003.
72. Fuks, A, Brawer J, Boudreau JD. The foundation of physicianship. *Perspect Biol Med*. 2017; 55(1):114–126.

Teaching the Social Sciences in Residency

ZAC FEILCHENFELD, AYELET KUPER,

FARAH FRIESEN, AMANDA CHEN,

AND CYNTHIA WHITEHEAD

Introduction

The social sciences are used to study human society, social organization, and other social phenomena. The term "social science" is used in contrast to the so-called natural sciences (such as biology, physics, chemistry, and mathematics and their subfields) and encompasses a vast array of disciplines, including sociology, economics, history, political science, and geography, among many others. Some of these disciplines may also be considered to be in the humanities (e.g., history).

The social sciences offer valuable ideas, concepts, perspectives, and theories that are essential to physician training. Social science education is particularly well-suited to graduate medical education. With the clinical experience of graduate trainees, the clinical relevance of social science concepts and ideas is easier to understand, and there would be greater capacity to generate discussion. The need for continuation of content is essential; a social science foundation in undergraduate medical education would set the stage for more advanced training. Just as basic science concepts are first encountered in medical school, those that become increasingly relevant need to be reviewed at a higher level (e.g., radiologists may review physics; nephrologists may review biochemistry). In this chapter, we begin by establishing the historical and contemporary contexts for integrating social science content in medical education and then examine the literature on the incorporation of social science knowledge in graduate medical education. We then discuss a conceptual model of the social science knowledge that underpins the non-Medical Expert Canadian Medical Education Directions for Specialists (CanMEDS) roles as an evidence-based foundation from which to develop seminars, courses, and curricula that involve the social sciences.

Social Sciences in Medical Education

Proposals to integrate social science content into medical education have a long history. As early as 1936, medical historian Henry Sigerist eloquently called on medical students to acquire some knowledge in the social sciences: "not to make you experts in the subject but you must have a certain knowledge in order to be able to understand the world in which you live."[1] In the postwar period, famed sociologist of medicine Albert F. Wessen noted "the sudden entry of the social sciences into the medical college" drawing parallels to the turn of the century movement to incorporate biological sciences into medical practice and education.[2] Barriers, however, were also identified early, including a crowded curriculum and students' perspectives with regards to the content's relevancy to their learning.[3,4] The introduction of a "biopsychosocial" model of disease, incorporating non-biomedical factors in the understanding of health and illness,[5] and the development of "behavioral sciences"[6] (at the outset described as "an amalgamation of sociology, cultural anthropology, social psychology, and clinical psychology"[7]) have made more lasting impacts on medical training.

Discussions of whether, how, and to what extent social sciences should be a part of medical education have continued.[8-10]

The past two decades have seen increased support from institutional authorities for the integration of social sciences (with emphasis on behavioral sciences) in medical education:

- A 2004 report by the Institute of Medicine (IOM) highlighted the importance of social and behavioral factors in health, described the history of approaches to incorporating social science content into curricula, and recommended curricular topics and strategies for the incorporation of these topics to enhance the social science education provided during medical school.[11]
- In 2011, the Association of American Medical Colleges (AAMC) published a report by an expert panel intended to improve the teaching of behavioral and social sciences in medical schools, incorporating the IOM report, the Accreditation Council for Graduate Medical Education (ACGME) core competencies and the CanMEDS roles (Box 6.1).[12]
- In the United Kingdom, the Behavioral and Social Sciences Teaching in Medicine network described the evolution of behavioral and social science education in British medical education in a 2010 report funded by the Higher Education Academy.[13]

A contemporary rationale provided for the incorporation of behavioral and social sciences teaching in medical education is the need for competency frameworks to ensure physicians are trained in all the skills necessary to improve and maintain patients' health. While the question of whether competency-based medical education (CBME) will achieve its aims remains to be answered, the current context of medical education in many countries requires educators and program directors to work within the CBME paradigm. Accordingly, education in the biomedical sciences, the traditional domain of medical knowledge, may not afford medical learners a foundation to support the full suite of competencies expected of a physician.[14]

BOX 6.1 North American Competency Frameworks

ACGME Core Competencies

Patient care
Medical knowledge
Practice-based learning and improvement
Interpersonal and communication skills
Professionalism
Systems-based practice

CanMEDS Roles

Medical expert
Communicator
Collaborator
Leader (formerly Manager)
Health advocate
Scholar
Professional

The institutional reports cited largely focus on the teaching of social sciences in undergraduate medical education. In this context, there seems to be a sufficient volume of literature to allow for a Best Evidence Medical Education Collaboration systematic review.[15] This review has not yet been published, but a recent update (August 23, 2016) indicated the identification of 81 relevant papers.[16] The importance of social science knowledge to medical school is also evident in the "elevation" of the social sciences to feature in the current iteration of the Medical College Admission Test entrance examination.[17,18] Medical schools that emphasize social science as a core discipline are leading calls for further reformation of undergraduate medical curricula to increase the attention to the social aspects of medicine in medical education.[19,20]

Uses of Social Sciences in Graduate Medical Education

As with the humanities, social sciences teaching in graduate medical education (residency training) is less well-established than in undergraduate medical curricula. We conducted a formal literature review of the use of social sciences in graduate medical education, exposing the paucity of dedicated social sciences teaching in residency. The disparity between teaching in social science and humanities topics in graduate compared with undergraduate medical education has been noted for decades. In 1984, Povar and Keith found that internal medicine residency program directors in the United States felt there was a need for more time and resources to be dedicated to incorporating essential "liberal arts subjects" into the graduate curriculum.[21]

Literature Search Approach

A trained librarian conducted a search to identify literature related to the *use of social sciences in graduate medical education*. PubMed and OVID Medline databases were searched from inception to August 15, 2016. Keywords and medical subject headings (MeSH) were combined to capture the concepts of social sciences and graduate medical education. Keywords included "medical education," "medical school," resident/s, residency, trainee*, postgraduate*, "junior doctor/s," "foundation doctor/s," "specialty registrar/s," "house officer/s," preceptor, preceptorship, "social science*," sociology, and anthropology and MeSH included Education, Medical, Graduate; Schools, Medical; Internship and residency; Preceptorship; Social sciences; Sociology; and Anthropology. Specific searches for psychology and political science did not produce additional results that were relevant to our literature search.

The results (n = 17,580) from PubMed and OVID Medline were imported into EndNote and de-duplicated (n = 3,415). A total of 14,165 titles and abstracts were reviewed for relevance (See Figure 6.1).

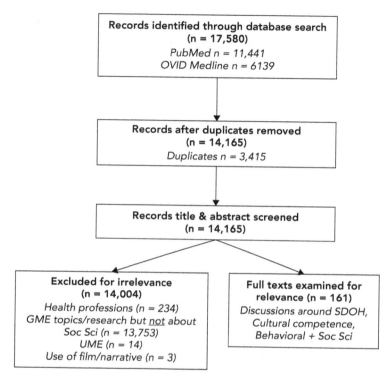

FIGURE 6.1. Literature search strategy conducted using PubMed and OVID Medline databases. GME = graduate medical education; Soc Sci = social sciences; UME = undergraduate medical education; SDOH = social determinants of health.

In addition, a search of grey literature (documents written and published outside of major distribution channels and often difficult to find in the most commonly consulted bibliographic databases [http://hlwiki.slais.ubc.ca/index.php/Grey_literature]) was undertaken using Google and Google Scholar. Keywords were searched, using combinations of: "behavioral science," "social science," teaching, medicine, "medical education," residency, resident, and curriculum. MedEdPortal® (www.mededportal.org AAMC; an online open-access publication of peer-reviewed health professions education materials) was searched for the terms (separately): "social science," sociology, and ethnography.

Findings

Our literature review, though systematic, does not purport to be comprehensive in scope.[22] Following literature review standards, the findings are presented narratively in the following sections, with select references representing the relevant themes identified through our search. Most of the records identified through our systematic search were deemed irrelevant; most often, articles were either related to social sciences topics, though not situated in graduate medical education, or related to graduate medical education topics unconnected to the social sciences.

Barriers

Barriers to further incorporation of social science topics in residency programs are no different than any other element of the curriculum, including pressures on curricular time, financial resources, faculty availability, and residents' competing interests. Since residency programs predominantly deliver educational content outside of a traditional classroom, it might be hoped that social science topics are regularly being encountered during workplace-based educational activities. Satterfield et al. evaluated the likelihood of discussion of social and behavioral science topics during hospital-based patient care rounds. They found that these topics arose in most patient encounters, some more frequently than others, but that "'teachable moments' are not being fully utilized."[23]

Behavioral and Social Sciences and Social Determinants of Health

The literature suggests that psychiatry programs are at the forefront of attempts to incorporate social sciences (as overlapping and intersecting disciplines) in residency training. In one example, Bromley and Braslow describe a series of modules incorporating tools and concepts from social sciences (including anthropology, sociology, and history) to help psychiatry residents develop critical skills.[24] The goals of this course include helping residents "Recognize the historical and cultural roots of clinical tools; Learn basic concepts, including reductionism and social construction; Think critically about received wisdom in psychiatry."[24] Another approach applies psychological and sociological theories to help psychiatry residents learn to reframe illness as a multifactorial process.[25]

Many texts describe the integration of two concepts that we feel can be best understood as instrumental applications of social science knowledge. These are the Behavioral and Social Sciences (BSS) and the Social Determinants of Health (SDOH) (Box 6.2 lists the general domains of BSS knowledge; Box 6.3 lists some of the SDOH, which are interrelated in complex systems, as described in detail in World Health Organization [WHO] publications[26,27]). We consider the uses of BSS and SDOH instrumental applications because trainees are not required to have any foundational social science knowledge prior to being taught this content. This does not preclude the utility of these concepts; by analogy, students can gain from lessons about clinical cardiology without any knowledge of cardiac physiology. Publications with curricula dedicated

---

BOX 6.2 General Domains of BSS Knowledge

- Mind-body interaction in health and disease
- Patient behavior
- Physician role and behavior
- Physician-patient interactions
- Social and cultural issues in healthcare
- Health policy and economics

> **BOX 6.3 Social Determinants of Health**
>
> - Socioeconomic and political context—including cultural norms and values, political stability, government policies
> - Social position—including educational status, income, gender, ethnicity
> - Psychosocial factors, behaviors, and biological factors

to improving students BSS skills explicitly adopt concepts from the IOM and AAMC documents highlighted in the first section of this chapter.[11,12] Curricula designed to improve students' understanding of SDOH use concepts and ideas defined by the WHO.[27]

We found examples of BSS curricular interventions predominantly in our search of grey literature. Satterfield and Carney summarize the efforts of medical schools organized in 2005 as the BSS Consortium for Medical Education, through which 16 medical schools created and implemented innovations in BSS curricula.[28] Teaching materials including a workshop designed to train clinical teachers to incorporate social and behavioral constructs into teaching, and a "Toolbox" of BSS "pearls" are available online (https://www.mededportal.org/).[29,30] Finally, Carney et al. conducted an extensive systematic review, identifying many validated measurement instruments for assessing general "BSS competencies."[31] These were defined by the authors as communication skills, cultural competence/patient-centered care competencies, empathy/compassion, behavioral health counseling competencies, professionalism competencies, and teamwork competencies.[31]

The conceptual framework of SDOH is a model of the complex influences of social, political, physical, material, and biological factors on health, healthcare, and well-being.[26] Chokshi argues for rearranging medical education around SDOH toward a more patient-centered and holistic curriculum, in contrast to the disease- or organ system-centered curriculum found in most medical schools.[32] Martinez et al. provide "twelve tips" for teaching SDOH in medical school, recommendations based on critical experience that can help guide adaptation to local educational contexts.[33] One medical school designed a curriculum to focus on social justice in hopes of "improv[ing] student recognition and rectification of adverse social determinants of disease."[34] The only source which describes SDOH being incorporated into a graduate curriculum employs an Entrustable Professional Activity (a construct used as part of a competency assessment) to assess pediatric residents' ability to manage SDOH.[35]

Competencies and Social Sciences

Residency programs are tasked with delivering curricula that produce physicians competent in aptitudes beyond biomedical knowledge. In the competency paradigm, programs in the United States are tasked with training physicians competent in "systems-based practices" (an abstract construct defined as the ability "to understand complex systems, navigate them for the benefit of patients, and lead or participate in continually improving them"[36]) and "professionalism"; in Canada and other jurisdictions that have adopted or adapted the CanMEDS framework, programs must train "health advocates" and "professionals."[37,38] However, there are well-established concerns with the validity and reliability of assessing the ACGME general competencies aside from Medical Knowledge,[39] and even the validity of the ACGME competencies as distinct and measurable constructs,[40] though these concerns are disputed.[41] Similarly, the teaching and assessment of CanMEDS roles aside from Medical Expert has been debated in the literature.[42-44] We take the approach that foundational social science knowledge is important to the practice of medicine, and we make use of competency frameworks as means with which such knowledge can be incorporated into medical education.

Knowledge from the social sciences is required to develop competency in at least some of the non-Medical Knowledge ACGME competencies and non-Medical Expert CanMEDS roles, despite the primary focus on biomedical science.[14] We highlight two clear intersections of prominent competency frameworks and the social sciences to examine the ways in which these topics are currently taught and assessed: advocacy education (providing learners with tools to harness their role as physicians to address determinants of health affecting patients as individuals and in communities) and the notion of "cultural competence" (largely enacted as the ability to interact with patients from different backgrounds without causing offense).

Arguing for increased advocacy training in undergraduate and graduate medical education, Croft et al. cite ACGME recommendations and make a case for such training using rationales based in professionalism and medical ethics.[45] Advocacy curricula range in scope. Daniels et al. describe a series of lectures provided to orthopedic surgery residents.[46] They found that the lectures increased residents' perspective of the importance of advocacy. In a larger project, Sharma describes an advocacy curriculum delivered to internal medicine residents integrated into the traditional educational program at one hospital.[47] More extensively, Martin et al. report on a two-year curriculum teaching health policy and health system-level advocacy to family medicine residents.[48] This curriculum was well-reviewed, and students' knowledge of health policy content improved. These advocacy curricula make use of social science concepts such as equity, culture, and identity formation, though the authors do not always explicitly identify the social science concepts used in their curricula.

The notion of "cultural competence" is a dominant frame for educational approaches that address cultural diversity and health inequities, though it has been criticized for "essentializing, commodifying, and appropriating culture, leading to stereotyping and further disempowerment of patients."[49] Determining how to incorporate cultural competence education into residency programs has been the subject of several publications. Chun et al. interviewed several educators in general surgery training programs who produced differing recommendations.[50] A similar study examining the approaches to teaching cultural competence among educators in psychiatry programs again yielded a range of suggested teaching methods.[51] One recommendation was to include faculty with training in social sciences or humanities. Much of the literature on cultural competence in graduate training relates to psychiatry. A detailed curriculum is described by Fung et al.[52] in which the authors heavily involved experts from social science disciplines in the creation and development of the course. Although many cultural competence curricula have been published and more have been implemented in undergraduate and residency programs, there is a lack of detailed qualitative analysis. Willen et al. conducted an anthropological study of one cultural competence curriculum in a psychiatry residency program.[53] Nuances related to residents' affective experiences of this course, the need for capacity and support for public and personal reflection, and a desire for case-based discussions that engage the residents are just some of the authors' insights. Lacking a foundation in the social sciences, these cultural competence curricula often boil down to memorization of facts about different cultures. Whereas the advocacy training programs based their curricula on core social science concepts, many of the published cultural competence curricula are quite simplified and disconnected from the highly relevant social science knowledge that could enrich these programs. In our view, education in cultural knowledge, supporting person-centered care, and cultural safety should be inextricable from social science concepts.[54]

Critique of Instrumental Approaches

Using instrumental applications of social science knowledge without providing a foundational social science education may not achieve the intended goals. One study evaluated a curriculum in which students were exposed to social justice topics described as "an amalgam of unrelated course material lacking sustained attention to crucial themes of power and powerlessness."[55] This course made no difference in students' social awareness, sensitivity to cultural and social diversity, awareness of their own privilege, or understanding of power relationships. Although students could identify social and cultural differences, their ability to appreciate the relevance of these differences in professional and healthcare contexts was limited.[55] Though residents could conceivably learn important content in clinical cardiology courses without a more basic science foundation, there are obvious advantages of a background in cardiac physiology and anatomy, and even some basic biology. And yet, residents are often exposed to applied or instrumental uses of social science knowledge and expected to develop complex skills such as cultural safety, without a similar social science foundation. Forward-looking programs may require even more complex understanding of social science concepts as we task future physicians with developing "structural" competence, identifying and addressing health inequities at a structural level.[56,57]

The instrumental approaches taken by the educational projects described in our literature review directly address their curricular topics at a clinical level but do not cover the supporting knowledge itself. We think that providing a foundational social science curriculum that supports the broader competencies expected of physicians in the dominant competency frameworks (i.e., the ACGME competencies outside of Medical Knowledge and the CanMEDS roles outside of Medical Expert) would be a valuable addition to medical training and would link the social sciences with the goals of competency frameworks.

Foundational Social Science Knowledge for Medical Training

Our literature review identifies several instrumental applications of social sciences in graduate medical education, though we could not find reports of dedicated uses of social science content to teach residents. This was not entirely surprising. With the ever-increasing growth of basic biomedical science content and clinical content in undergraduate and graduate training, there has historically been limited space in the curriculum for non-bioscientific knowledge.[58] And would the addition of social science training in medical school and residency necessarily create better physicians? In a commentary, one of the authors of this chapter questioned whether merely adding social science as an additional "ingredient" in medical training would produce the intended results.[59] Success would be unlikely without acknowledging dominant and highly valued forms of knowledge in medicine, nor without confronting changing paradigms in medical education (i.e., competency frameworks).

Identifying the non-bioscientific knowledge that underpins these broader competencies is the first step, and four of the authors of this chapter have been involved over the past several years in a project to do just that.[60] This project used the CanMEDS framework as we are based in Canada, but the results are likely transferable to other competency frameworks that incorporate competencies, skills, or traits beyond medical knowledge, such as the ACGME competencies. Academics from social science and humanities disciplines were interviewed to identify the forms of knowledge, theories, and facts within their disciplines that would support the development of competence in non-Medical Expert CanMEDS roles, leading to the formulation of a conceptual model (see Figure 6.2). This model is perhaps a more complex articulation than many teachers and program directors would be interested in applying to their programs without further involvement of content experts. Our literature review did not reveal any other models of the social science knowledge base that supports physician competencies that have been discussed or published. We suggest that this model, explained in detail in the full publication, can be adapted to cover the core content to which residents should be exposed. See Box 6.4 for discussion questions that highlight the relevance of social science knowledge for each of the non-Medical Expert CanMEDS roles.

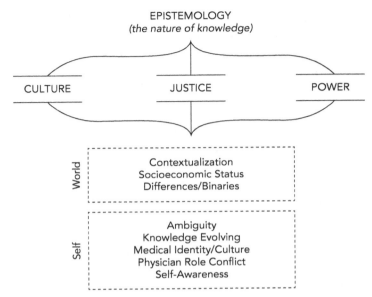

EPISTEMOLOGY
(the nature of knowledge)

CULTURE   JUSTICE   POWER

World

Contextualization
Socioeconomic Status
Differences/Binaries

Self

Ambiguity
Knowledge Evolving
Medical Identity/Culture
Physician Role Conflict
Self-Awareness

FIGURE 6.2. This model, derived from research findings, displays the cross-cutting themes encompassing the forms of knowledge, theories, and facts from domains outside of bioscience needed in the medical curricula to best support the training of physicians to be fully competent in the six non-Medical Expert CanMEDS roles. The model is constructed in a hierarchical manner, with epistemology as the foundational concept, necessary to a curriculum that grounds physician competencies in the social sciences. Next in the hierarchy are the anchoring themes of culture, justice, and power, which underpin all of the non-Medical Expert CanMEDS roles. These anchoring concepts link to the cross-cutting themes relating to a physician's relationships with the world and the self, each of which relates to differing degrees with the different CanMEDS roles. For further explanation, see the source article and the associated online appendix. Used with permission.[60]

Curricular Implementation

In the academic year 2015–2016, we initiated curricular projects piloting the implementation of educational materials based on our conceptual model in a small number of graduate programs within

BOX 6.4 Discussion Questions Linking Social Science Knowledge to the Non-Medical Expert CanMEDS Roles, with Example Themes to Explore

- Collaborator—What is the basis of power hierarchies in the clinical environment (e.g., between nurses, physicians, allied health personnel)? (Power, Socioeconomic Status, Self-awareness)
- Communicator—Though physicians aspire to provide culturally safe care, who should decide whether the care provided to a patient was safe? (Culture, Justice, Contextualization, Differences/Binaries)
- Health Advocate—From whose authority should a physician act as an advocate for a marginalized community? (Power, Justice, Physician Role Conflict)
- Leader/Manager—How can individual physicians justly allocate (or decline to allocate) finite health care resources for their patients? (Justice, Socioeconomic Status, Physician Role Conflict)
- Professional—What does it mean to be a *good doctor*, and how is that meaning developed? (Culture, Knowledge Evolving, Medical Identity/Culture, Self-Awareness)
- Scholar—What counts as evidence? (Alternatively, what constitutes legitimate knowledge?) (Epistemology, Ambiguity, Knowledge Evolving)

the Department of Medicine at the University of Toronto. These educational materials were individualized in consultation with graduate program directors to address the focused needs of each program to teach non-Medical Expert CanMEDS roles. The level of interest in the pilot program superseded our expectations, perhaps indicating program directors' perceptions of a lack of available alternatives. We worked with five graduate training programs, and we had to turn down four more program directors who wanted to be part of our pilot.

We consulted with each of the five involved programs to determine the material to be covered and the time available in the curriculum. One of the programs had a pre-existing curriculum designed to teach residents about the health advocate role through an advocacy project. The program director wanted to strengthen the theoretical underpinnings of this curriculum through integrating material from our conceptual model. Two other subspecialty programs chose to join the resulting two-session health advocate curriculum. One program director asked for a single session centered on the communicator role, with emphasis on communication across cultural and socioeconomic groups. The final program director had a similar interest in providing teaching in culturally safe communication and could arrange for three half-day sessions of curricular time (see sample curricula referenced in the website at the end of the chapter for adapted examples).

Lessons Learned in our Experiences with Implementation

We found the need to deliver similar basic concepts related to the foundational and anchoring themes of our conceptual model (epistemology, culture, justice, and power) despite the "focus" on different CanMEDS roles. With more curricular time available, we could give more attention to selected themes as they relate to each non-Medical Expert CanMEDS role. While we hope that the foundational and anchoring concepts will become increasingly familiar to residents if covered during undergraduate training, we expect that we will need to review the core ideas with future iterations of these curricula for some time.

Faculty involvement is necessary for the success of these curricula by underscoring the importance and legitimacy of this knowledge. However, finding clinical faculty who have sufficient knowledge and familiarity to teach this material can be challenging. We did not involve nonclinical teachers (i.e., social scientists), though this could

> **BOX 6.5 Building Capacity in Residents and Faculty to Teach Social Sciences**
>
> - Challenge: a lack of clinicians/educators with adequate training
> - Challenge: Departments and faculties may not value or recognize academic contributions of clinicians and educators with social science background
> - Solution: a dedicated, adequately trained small group of individuals to champion the inclusion of social sciences, provide a lot of faculty development, and encourage recruitment and promotion

certainly be explored. The small cadre of physicians in our department with graduate degrees in the social sciences were eager to participate in teaching this material. Faculty development and/or recruitment of faculty with backgrounds in the social sciences or humanities will be necessary for growth (see Box 6.5).

Finally, we found that being bound by the time constraints of as few as one half-day session limited the ability to cover enough material. The scant time allocation reflects the relative position of the non-Medical Expert CanMEDS roles (as compared with more traditional clinical content) in most curricula. However, considering our well-received pilot implementation, we have been offered increased teaching time in the future, including seven sessions over the three years of the core internal medicine program beginning in 2017–2018.

Summary

Physician training requires a broader education than can be offered by biomedical sciences alone.[14] Despite the current paradigm of

CBME with the recognition, at least in name, of physician roles beyond Medical Expert, the social science foundations of the non-Medical Expert roles (and similar constructs in other competency frameworks than CanMEDS) are seldom mentioned in the literature. Knowledge from the social sciences is steadily being integrated across the medical education continuum, though this content is not always explicitly labeled as social science. Concepts such as advocacy, professionalism, and cultural knowledge, embedded in competency frameworks such as CanMEDS and ACGME, are seldom discussed or taught beginning with foundational social science topics.

We find that the social sciences are most commonly incorporated into medical school curricula and residency programs through instrumental applications. These include curricula developed around the paradigms of BSS and SDOH, as well as specific competencies derived from competency frameworks, such as advocacy and cultural competence. Our critique of these instrumental approaches holds that foundational social science knowledge, as important as foundational basic science knowledge to clinical topics, is missing from the broader medical curriculum.

We present one approach, developed in recent years at the University of Toronto, to define core content derived from the social sciences that supports the non-Medical Expert CanMEDS roles. The themes and concepts are complex, which requires time to be devoted to teaching and learning this material. The complexity also allows for flexibility, so that the same core concepts are used toward different ends. Our experience illustrates this complexity and flexibility, demonstrates the interest of program directors and residents, and can serve as examples of how to design and implement theoretically-grounded curricula using social sciences in graduate medical education. In the appendix, we have referenced sample curricula, and in Box 6.6, five ideas that program directors could consider exploring more completely.

A sample curriculum to accompany this chapter can be found online at http://cahh.ca/resources/ouplesson-plans/.

BOX 6.6 Five Ideas to Consider for Graduate
Medical Education Seminars Incorporating
Social Science Knowledge

1. Social construction of knowledge—Epistemology, Ambiguity, Knowledge Evolving

   The Savvy Patient: Patients have access to medical information on the Internet (of uncertain quality). Physicians' approach to this extremely common occurrence may benefit from a broader perspective of knowledge creation than the traditional scientific model.

2. Patient narratives—Epistemology, Culture, Contextualization

   It's All History: Reality is contextual. Patients' experiences of health and illness, and their ability to communicate these experiences, are not uniform. Physicians' appreciation of the impact of lived experience and cultural (and socioeconomic, etc.) context on patients' narratives is necessary for good relationships and high quality care.

3. Cultural safety—Culture, Socioeconomic status, Differences/Binaries, Self-awareness

   She Just Doesn't Like Me: Physicians must do more than simply memorize the words and actions to avoid so as not to offend a patient from an "other" group (culture, gender, sexual orientation, etc.). Physicians-in-training can develop skills in self-reflection (exploring their own beliefs and actions) and reflexivity (exploring their own privileges, context/culture/history) to nurture humility in their interactions with marginalized patients.

4. Medical socialization—Power, Medical Identity/Culture, Self-awareness

"Doctor Important": Physicians hold a position of authority in healthcare micro-cultures and in society at large. This has effects on collaborative work, advocacy activities, and professional identity, among others. Physicians-in-training may benefit from a greater awareness of the effects of their socialization within medicine and from critical reflection about the powerful position they occupy as physicians.

5. Professional identity—Justice, Medical Identity/Culture, Physician Role Conflict

Lunch is Sponsored By . . . Physicians, as social actors, have obligations to their patients, society, themselves, their employers, their families, their debtors, and likely many other parties. Exploration of ethical frameworks and moral theories can help physicians-in-training navigate the conflicting demands on their time and integrity.

References

1. Sigerist HE. The medical student and the social problems confronting medicine today. *Bull Hist Med.* 1936; 4:411.
2. Wessen AF. Medical schools and the sociologist. *The Midwest Sociologist.* 1959; 21(2):77–85.
3. Hayes DP, Jackson JK. Teaching social science in the medical school: A case study in teamwork and practice. *J Health Hum Behav.* 1960; 1(1):34–41.
4. New PK-M, May JT. Teaching activities of social scientists in medical and public health schools. *Soc Sci Med.* 1968; 2(4):447–460.
5. Engel GL. The need for a new medical model: A challenge for biomedicine. *Science.* 1977; 196(4286):129–136.

6. Coe RM. Teaching behavioral sciences in schools of medicine: Observations on some Latin-American schools. *Soc Sci Med.* 1975;9(4–5):221–225.doi:10.1016/0037-7856(75)90025–90026

7. West LJ. Behavioral sciences in the medical school curriculum. *Acad Med.* 1959; 34(11):1070–1076.

8. Begun JW, Rieker PP. Social science in medicine: the question of "relevance." *Acad Med.* 1980; 55(3):181–185.

9. MacLeod S, McCullough H. Social science education as a component of medical training. *Soc Sci Med.* 1994; 39(9):1367–1373.

10. Whitehead C. Scientist or science-stuffed? Discourses of science in North American medical education. *Med Educ.* 2013; 47(1):26–32.

11. Cuff PA, Vanselow N. *Improving medical education: Enhancing the behavioral and social science content of medical school curricula.* Washington, DC: National Academies Press; 2004.

12. Charon R, Holmboe E, Holmes JH, et al. Behavioral and Social Science Foundations for Future Physicians: Report of the Behavioral and Social Science Expert Panel. https://www.aamc.org/download/271020/data/behavioralandsocialsciencefoundationsforfuturephysicians.pdf Published November 2011. Accessed October 19, 2016.

13. Bundy C, Cordingley L, Peters S, Rock J, Hart J, Hodges L. A Core Curriculum for Psychology in Undergraduate Medical Education. https://www.heacademy.ac.uk/system/files/core-curriculum-for-psychology-undergrad-medical-education.pdf Published 2010. Accessed October 19, 2016.

14. Kuper A, D'Eon M. Rethinking the basis of medical knowledge. *Med Educ.* 2011; 45(1):36–43.

15. Hothersall EJ, Harden J, Fioratou E, Manca A, Gordon M, Schofield S. Protocol: Assessing the behavioural and social science curricular components for undergraduate medical students: A BEME systematic review. http://bemecollaboration.org/downloads/2472/Protocol%20Jan%20(2016).pdf Published January 10 2016. Accessed October 19, 2016.

16. Hothersall EJ. Project update: Assessing the behavioural and social science curricula components for undergraduate medical students: A BEME systematic review. http://bemecollaboration.org/downloads/2658/Project%20Update%20August%202016.pdf. Published August 23, 2016. Accessed October 19, 2016.

17. Louie LRA, Bereknyei MGS. Elevating the behavioral and social sciences in premedical training: MCAT2015. *Acad Psychiatry* 2015; 39:127–131.

18. Kaplan RM, Satterfield JM, Kington RS. Building a better physician—The case for the new MCAT. *N Engl J Med.* 2012; 366(14):1265–1268.

19. Kasper J, Greene JA, Farmer PE, Jones DS. All health is global health, all medicine is social medicine: Integrating the social sciences into the preclinical curriculum. *Acad Med.* 2016; 91(5):628–632

20. Westerhaus M, Finnegan A, Haidar M, Kleinman A, Mukherjee J, Farmer P. The necessity of social medicine in medical education. *Acad Med.* 2015; 90(5):565–568 doi: 10.1097/acm. 0000000000000571

21. Povar GJ, Keith KJ. The teaching of liberal arts in internal medicine residency training. *Acad Med.* 1984; 59(9):714–721

22. Grant MJ, Booth A. A typology of reviews: An analysis of 14 review types and associated methodologies. *Health Info Libr J.* 2009; 26(2):91–108.

23. Satterfield JM, Bereknyei S, Hilton JF, et al. The prevalence of social and behavioral topics and related educational opportunities during attending rounds. *Acad Med.* 2014; 89(11):1548–1557.

24. Bromley E, Braslow JT. Teaching critical thinking in psychiatric training: A role for the social sciences. *Am J Psychiatry.* 2008; 165(11):1396–1401 doi: 10.1176/appi.ajp.2008.08050690

25. Bolton JW. How to integrate biological, psychological, and sociological knowledge in psychiatric education: A case formulation seminar series. *Acad Psych.* 2015; 39(6):699–702.

26. Solar O, Irwin A. A Conceptual Framework for Action on the Social Determinants of Health. Social Determinants of Health Discussion Paper 2 (Policy and Practice) http://www.who.int/ social_determinants/corner/SDHDP2.pdf Published 2010. Accessed November 1, 2016.

27. Marmot M, Friel S, Bell R, Houweling TA, Taylor S, WHO Commission on Social Determinants of Health. Closing the gap in a generation: health equity through action on the social determinants of health. *The Lancet.* 2008; 372(9650):1661–1669.

28. Satterfield JM, Carney PA. Aligning Medical Education with the Nation's Health Priorities: Innovations in Physician Training in Behavioral and Social Sciences. http://www.ahrq.gov/

professionals/education/curriculum-tools/population-health/satterfield.html Published 2015. Accessed November 1, 2016.

29. Ramos JS, Bogetz AL, Bereknyei Merrell S, et al. Enhancing behavioral and social science at the bedside: Core skills for clinicians and teachers. MedEdPORTAL Publications. 2015; 11:10032 https://www.mededportal.org/publication/10032. Accessed November 1, 2016.

30. Saba G, Satterfield J, Salazar R, et al. The SBS toolbox: Clinical pearls from the social and behavioral sciences. MedEdPORTAL Publications. 2010; 6:7980. http://doi.org/10.15766/mep_2374-8265.7980. Accessed November 1, 2016.

31. Carney PA, Palmer RT, Miller MF, et al. Tools to assess behavioral and social science competencies in medical education: A systematic review. *Acad Med*. 2016; 91(5):730–742.

32. Chokshi DA. Teaching about health disparities using a social determinants framework. *J Gen Intern Med*. 2010; 25(2):182–185.

33. Martinez IL, Artze-Vega I, Wells AL, Mora JC, Gillis M. Twelve tips for teaching social determinants of health in medicine. *Med Teach*. 2015; 37(7):647–652.

34. Coria A, McKelvey TG, Charlton P, Woodworth M, Lahey T. The design of a medical school social justice curriculum. *Acad Med*. 2013; 88(10):1442–1449.

35. Klein MD, Schumacher DJ, Sandel M. Assessing and managing the social determinants of health: Defining an entrustable professional activity to assess residents' ability to meet societal needs. *Acad Pediatr*. 2014; 14(1):10–13.

36. Guralnick S, Ludwig S, Englander R. Domain of competence: Systems-based practice. *Acad Pediatr*. 2014; 14(2):S70–S79 doi: 10.1016/j.acap.2013.11.015

37. ACGME. Common Program Requirements. https://www.acgme.org/Portals/0/PFAssets/ProgramRequirements/CPRs_07012016.pdf. Updated September 28, 2014. Accessed November 4, 2016.

38. Frank JR, Snell L, Sherbino J, eds. *CanMEDS 2015 Physician Competency Framework*. Ottawa: Royal College of Physicians and Surgeons of Canada, 2015.

39. Lurie SJ, Mooney CJ, Lyness JM. Measurement of the general competencies of the Accreditation Council for Graduate Medical Education: A systematic review. *Acad Med*. 2009; 84(3):301–309.

40. Lurie SJ, Mooney CJ, Lyness JM. Commentary: Pitfalls in assessment of competency-based educational objectives. *Acad Med*. 2011; 86(4):412–414.

41. Green ML, Holmboe E. Perspective: the ACGME toolbox: Half empty or half full? *Acad Med*. 2010; 85(5):787–790.

42. Chou S, Cole G, McLaughlin K, Lockyer J. CanMEDS evaluation in Canadian postgraduate training programmes: Tools used and programme director satisfaction. *Med Educ*. 2008; 42(9):879–886 doi: 10.1111/j.1365-2923.2008.03111.x

43. Verma S, Flynn L, Seguin R. Faculty's and residents' perceptions of teaching and evaluating the role of health advocate: A study at one Canadian university. *Acad Med*. 2005; 80(1):103–108.

44. Whitehead CR, Kuper A, Hodges B, Ellaway R. Conceptual and practical challenges in the assessment of physician competencies. *Med Teach*. 2015; 37(3):245–251.

45. Croft D, Jay SJ, Meslin EM, Gaffney MM, Odell JD. Perspective: Is it time for advocacy training in medical education? *Acad Med*. 2012; 87(9):1165–1170.

46. Daniels AH, Bariteau JT, Grabel Z, DiGiovanni CW. Prospective analysis of a novel orthopedic residency advocacy education program. *R I Med J*. 2014; 97(10):43–46.

47. Sharma M. Developing an integrated curriculum on the health of marginalized populations: Successes, challenges, and next steps. *J Health Care Poor Underserved*. 2014; 25(2):663–669 doi: 10.1353/hpu.2014.0102

48. Martin D, Hum S, Han M, Whitehead C. Laying the foundation: Teaching policy and advocacy to medical trainees. *Med Teach*. 2013; 35(5):352–358 doi: 10.3109/0142159x.2013.770453

49. Kirmayer LJ. Rethinking cultural competence. *Transcult Psychiatry*. 2012;49(2):149–164 doi:10.1177/1363461512444673

50. Chun MB, Young KG, Jackson DS. Incorporating cultural competency into the general surgery residency curriculum: A preliminary assessment. *Int J Surg*. 2009; 7(4):368–372.

51. Hansen H, Dugan TM, Becker AE, et al. Educating psychiatry residents about cultural aspects of care: A qualitative study of approaches used by US expert faculty. *Acad Psych*. 2013; 37(6):412–416.

52. Fung K, Andermann L, Zaretsky A, Lo H-T. An integrative approach to cultural competence in the psychiatric curriculum. *Acad Psych*. 2008; 32(4):272–282.

53. Willen SS, Bullon A, Good M-JD. Opening up a huge can of worms: Reflections on a "cultural sensitivity" course for psychiatry residents. *Harv Rev Psychiatry*. 2010; 18(4):247–253.

54. Kuper A. When I say . . . cultural knowledge. *Med Educ*. 2014; 48(12):1148–1149.

55. Beagan BL. Teaching social and cultural awareness to medical students: "It's all very nice to talk about it in theory, but ultimately it makes no difference." *Acad Med.* 2003; 78(6):605–614.

56. Metzl JM, Hansen H. Structural competency: Theorizing a new medical engagement with stigma and inequality. *Soc Sci Med.* 2014; 103:126–133.

57. Bourgois P, Holmes S, Sue K, Quesada J. Structural vulnerability: Operationalizing the concept to address health disparities in clinical care. *Acad Med.* 2017; 92(3):299–307.

58. Sales CS, Schlaff AL. Reforming medical education: A response to Weller and Woodward, and Whitehead, and Schwab. *Soc Sci Med.* 2010; 70(11):1680–1681.

59. Whitehead C. Recipes for medical education reform: Will different ingredients create better doctors? A commentary on Sales and Schlaff. *Soc Sci Med.* 2010; 70(11):1672–1676 doi: 10.1016/j.socscimed.2010.02.017

60. Kuper A, Veinot P, Leavitt J, et al. Epistemology, culture, justice & power: Non-bioscientific knowledge for medical training. *Med Educ.* 2017;51(2):158–173 doi: doi:10.1111/medu.13115

The Use of Theater with Medical Residents

An Embodied Approach to Learning about Self and Other

L. J. NELLES, PEGGY HAMILTON,

PAUL ROBERT D'ALESSANDRO,

JEREMY REZMOVITZ, LU GAO,

SUVENDRINI LENA, AND ANNA SKORZEWSKA

"I regard the theatre as the greatest of all art forms, the most immediate way in which a human being can share with another the sense of what it is to be a human being."
— OSCAR WILDE

Introduction

Theater is indeed multiple. As story or spectacle it offers infinite ways of seeing and being, but, perhaps most importantly, as Wilde suggests, it illuminates the human condition. The multiperspectival capacity of theater offers medical residents a vehicle to engage with complex stories, ethical dilemmas, ambiguity, and themes which are intricately woven into the fabric of medical practice. Theater, through plays or performances, can tell stories that frame multiple perspectives at once and capture the complexity of lived experience. There are a myriad of ways in which theater or performance practice can be used as a teaching tool with residents. Experiential workshops teach residents about self and other, create meaning from experience, and develop self-awareness that is particularly useful at the point in their career where their responsibilities as working physicians increase. Through immediate engagement, residents examine perspective, ethics, biases, assumptions, and positionality and thus may develop a capacity for reflection, attunement, cooperation, and empathy, all of which comprise elements of expected professional competencies. To provide context for understanding the mechanisms through which theater and/or performance is thought to elicit change, this chapter is set within a performance studies paradigm. It provides a broad focus on the use of theater in the education of medical residents with examples of how it is being used with this population internationally and with a specific focus on four interventions that use theater differently in Canada. The first project "Ed's Story: the Dragon Chronicles" by D'Alessandro, Butterworth, and Frager is an example of theater in research. In this project a verbatim play about the lived experience of illness and end of life was shown to first-year medical students from the University of British Columbia. Verbatim theater is a genre that uses the words of people taken from research interviews or life events and weaves them into a play. The project examined the effects of the play on the students and mapped the results directly to Canadian Medical Education Directions for Specialists (CanMEDS) roles, the competencies required in Canadian residency training and which include communication, collaboration, professionalism, and advocacy. The second project details the work of neurologist and playwright Suvendrini Lena, who uses writing and performance as tools with residents to enhance their understanding of self and the perspective of other. In these workshops, residents read quality works of theater that contain medical content and, with the assistance of professional artists, do their own writing and performances. The third and fourth projects use aspects of performance or actor training in workshops that develop self-awareness, keen observation, deep listening, and an embodied ability to be fully present and responsive in the moment. Psychiatrist (and co-editor of this book) Anna Skorzewska has offered a series of arts-based seminars to psychiatry residents for five years. The theater seminars focus on performance and the body and are led by a professional actor. The final project by Drs. Jeremy Rezmovitz and Lu Gao at the University of Toronto provides improvisation workshops to students and residents. Improvisation, or improv, is a performance practice in which participants create scenes or skits in the moment; some well-known examples of this genre are found on *Saturday Night Live* and *Second City TV*. These workshops are based on bioethics and humanities professor, and *Second City* faculty, Katie Watson's 10-hour "Medical Improv" course. The goals of the course include enhanced "on the spot" communication, thinking, listening, and collaboration.[1] Here too the project leaders have found that skills learned through the improv workshop can be mapped onto medical competencies. Each of these projects will be examined in this chapter with a brief overview of current literature on interventions that use theater with residents. Authors of the chapter were approached by the lead author (LJN) due to their experience using theater with residents. Authors were asked to describe their programs, and follow-up interviews probed more fully their rationale for using theater, their lived experiences in using theater with residents, and their own backgrounds in theater/performance. These interviews were carried out by a professional actor and medical student (PH). Additionally, the experience of the lead author as actor, scholar, and arts educator provided sources germane to the theoretical performance frame. Resources to aid in program development can be found in the appendix.

Why Use Theater in the Education of Residents?

In his work on patient encounters, Elliot Mishler proposed that there are two distinct worlds trying to communicate in healthcare interactions. One voice represents the patient's life and experience, and one represents the medical world. He points out that there is a "struggle between the 'voice of the life world' and the 'voice of medicine' [where] in a typical medical encounter the voice of the life world tends to be suppressed in favor of the voice of medicine."[2] This chapter proposes that using theater with medical residents may be a way to allow the "voice of the life world" to be heard. Performance scholar, critical ethnographer, and activist Dwight Conquergood was instrumental in promoting performance as a paradigm for understanding the human condition. He saw performance as both a lens for understanding and a mechanism for change. Conquergood's suggestion of the "epistemological potential of performance as a way of deeply sensing the other" continues to propel the work of performance scholars, anthropologists, and ethnographers and underlines the value of using theater as an educational tool. Theater and medicine are rigorous practices. Actors integrate elements of their craft through hours of physical practice and self-reflection and, as a result, learn to see and be seen. They develop a language with which to describe the metaphoric landscape of the body and gain the ability to deeply sense and understand the other through performance.[3] Artist and performance scholar Warren Linds suggests that metaxis (defined by Plato as a place of "in between") allows us to simultaneously inhabit two worlds at the same time (in this case self and other). He offers: "through metaxic action, our bodies become generative sites of knowing."[4] Bringing theater practice to medical education offers residents an opportunity to develop the body as a site of knowledge. The acute awareness of self and other required of residents may not have been developed through traditional undergraduate communication skills teaching. In an examination of communication and relationship in medical practice, Zoppi and Epstein propose that communication is comprised of obtainable skills and a form of deep sensing they refer to as "being in relation with."[5] They suggest that this capacity can be developed through actor training methods. While there is evidence to support that some elements of communication can be taught, it has also been found that empathy can diminish over time,[6] perhaps because the body of the practitioner is often left out of this training. Professor of medical ethics and humanities Gretchen Case and physician Daniel Brauner propose using a performance studies paradigm that incorporates actor training methods in communication teaching. They suggest that this would develop a more embodied understanding of empathic imagination or "thinking with the other by thinking as the other"[7] and promote the reflection and analysis of both performance and human interaction. Other authors whose work corroborates the value of using performance methods in medical education to these ends include Anne de la Croix et al.,[8] Martin Kohn,[9] Melissa McCullough,[10] Yolanda Waslenko,[11] and Suzy Willson.[12]

Literature Search

This literature search contains two sections. The first is a short review of performance theory that supports the use of performance practice to teach embodied practice and critical thinking. The second details a brief review of theater in medical education literature. The search for this was carried out on PubMed, JSTOR, and the University of Manitoba database using the keywords theater, performance, medical residents, and education. Of the resulting 62 papers, 8 were relevant, as the word "theater" in the majority of papers referred to the operating theater. Removing the word "resident" provided the same results. A broad approach was subsequently used with only the words "theater" and "health." This resulted in 1,977 results. Filtering out papers that used theater to mean surgery and any projects not directly related to medical education resulted in a total of 47 results, 32 of which were deemed directly relevant to this chapter.

Although not all papers concerned medical residents, the results could be extrapolated to be relevant. The papers had a variety of theoretical frameworks and methodologies that were sometimes reflected by the background of the researchers/authors. While much of the literature regarding the use of theater in medical education focuses on programs directed at medical students rather than residents, many of the arguments for using theater at the undergraduate level can be applied to residents or other clinical professions; where this is true the literature was included in this chapter. Additionally it is important to note that those who use performance-based practice as a teaching tool are also privy to the benefits to learners. They witness the transformation as learners develop self-awareness and grow more confident and expressive.

However, it is a challenge to measure the effects or intended outcomes of using theater as a teaching tool because it is multifactorial and therefore difficult to know the precise factors that affect change when change is perceived to occur. Thus, much of the literature is not evidence in an empirical/quantitative way but is more often qualitative or theoretical in nature. In an age of evidence-based education this can create obstacles to funding theater-based curricula. An important consideration as postgraduate medicine seeks to build an evidence base for theater in education is that we may have to develop new methods of evaluation to capture the complex phenomena at play in theater-based activities. A scoping review on arts-based research in health by Boydell et al. suggests that "the growing use of arts-based knowledge creation and dissemination strategies is driving an important shift in our understanding of what counts as evidence, as well as appreciation for the complexity and multidimensionality involved in creating new knowledge."[13] Research methods in arts-based research are often quite different from those in medical education research and can offer a rich understanding of data that quantitative evidence based methods, while important, do not always capture. As far back as 2000, Delese Wear and Brian Castellani called for changes to health professions curricula that would see medical schools move away from strictly biomedical knowledge to the kind of knowledge that promotes other ways of thinking. They suggested that "real knowledge"—scientific—is gained through rational inquiry that is characterized by objectivity, universality, and replicability even though individuality and subjectivity have much to do with the experience of illness.[14] Medical humanities professor Martin Kohn suggests that humanities in medicine programs have an opportunity through theater to bridge the gaps between arts and medicine through the provision of different ways of knowing. He sees medical education as a moral enterprise where doctors need to learn to do the right thing under duress and suggests that theater-based curricula can facilitate this. Kohn insists that there should be sound research attached to these endeavors and, while he understands the value and need for "irreducible" quantitative knowledge in science, he suggests that reducing theater to measurable components may not be worth the small amount of "respectability" it would bring. Echoing Boydell, he proposes that rich collaborative qualitative arts-informed methods will have broader impact.[15]

In order to understand how theater evokes change, it is important to note that developments in neuroscience can provide an understanding of the internal mechanisms at play in performance training. In "Falsifiable Theories for Theatre and Performance Studies," McConachie outlines this turn away from a semiotic and discursive understanding of theater and toward a phenomenological and neuroscientific frame based on the work of scientists such as Damasio[16] and Neiderthal[17](embodied emotion), Gallese[18] and Iacoboni[19](mirror neurons), Coliani[20] (social cognition) and others.[21] This neuroscientific lens has had a parallel impact on other fields such as mindfulness, trauma-informed therapy,[22] and social cognition.[23] Vital to this discussion is the way that cognitive processes illuminate how performance works to influence individual change and empathy. In *Embodied Acting*, actor and performance scholar Rick Kemp shows that physiologist Vittorio Gallese's work on mirror neuron systems can illuminate the phenomenon of emotional responses to characters on a stage. He states that "visual information about the emotions of others is directly mapped onto the same viscero-motor neural structures that determine the experience of that emotion in the observer. This direct mapping can occur even when the emotion of others can only be imagined."[24] Theater director and scholar Amy Cook who specializes in the intersections of neuroscience and theater uses Gallese's work to connect the mirror neuron system to performance and empathy using his theory of intentional attunement. Quoting Gallese she explains intentional attunement as "the direct experience of what another is experiencing" which he calls "embodied simulation"; this allows the subject to feel "as if" he or she were doing what the observed was doing. This transfers perspective to a neural level, since doing the action recalls the intentions necessary for such actions and creates a kind of union or attunement.[25] In both medicine and theater, one might suggest that embodied presence manifests as attunement, and, as neuroscience suggests, knowledge can be generated from the body rather than only through the traditional paths of observation and analysis and that the use of theater with residents should generate some degree of embodied knowing, presence, and attunement.

Storytelling and Research

Most commonly, theater is used to tell stories, to present social and political issues in healthcare, or as a means of knowledge translation by health researchers. In Canada, playwrights work with researchers (Julia Gray *After the Crash*[26]) or create auto-ethnographic plays based on their own illness experience (Julie Devaney-*My Leaky Body*[27]), and researchers use arts-based practices to examine issues such as person-centered care in dementia (Kontos et al.)[28] or teen mental health (Boydell et al.).[29] One two-week program conducted by Jeffry et al. used drama educators and a palliative care physician to look at Pinter's *The Caretaker*. The program found it to be effective in addressing reflection and teamwork in end-of-life care that led to the discussion of themes of power, ethics, and communication.[30] Although used with medical students, this format and content could also be used with residents. Commercially successful plays such as *Wit, Angels in America, The Normal Heart,* and *Next to Normal* are all examples of work that feature the illness experience as a central theme. These and other plays that examine illness and the human condition offer a traditional use of theater as an artifact or educational tool to engage the student as witness in a particular topic. The UCLA medical school developed a standardized Reader's Theater activity using Margaret Edson's play *Wit*, which has been used throughout the United States and Canada. In Reader's Theater, learners read the script of a play out loud and then discuss the content of the play and the experience of being "other" through reading the characters in the play. *Wit* deals with complex communication and ethical issues through the story of one woman's experience of cancer. The play is often used for medical Reader's Theater and encourages reflection on advance care directives, empathy, breaking bad news, pain management, human suffering, and caring.[31] Performance scholar Kate Rossiter promotes the use of theater in medical education, suggesting that it fosters reflection on interrelational ethics and humanity. She proposes that the witty and unsentimental nature of *Wit* provides an excellent opportunity for this.[32] Medical Reader's Theater is a popular and cost-effective way to integrate theater into the medical curriculum. It allows students to "step into the skin of another" to foster reflection, dialogue, and understanding. A University of Michigan Reader's Theater program for family medicine residents uses an adaptation of *The Wizard of Oz* to examine medical ethics in which Dorothy is the patient, the witch cancer, and Oz the doctor. After learning about moral frameworks of power, the residents watch a scene from the film and read the adapted script together. Discussion is prompted by a series of questions that encourage a rich discussion about the ethics of power, institutions, and the complex relationships between characters. Residents evaluate this session highly and find it an effective way to apply the theoretical knowledge of ethics to practice.[33]

Finally, residents can participate in the creation of a play through the process of Devised Theater. Devised Theater encompasses a variety of genres. In many cases, a play is devised by the company around a particular theme, event, or issue without a central playwright. Sometimes a well-known piece is used as a central text and a new piece devised from it. Melissa McCullough has used this process successfully with students and residents and finds it particularly useful for examining complex ethical issues. She has learned through creating devised pieces with trainees that "medicine is not rigid and certain, that open-mindedness to the human condition is essential alongside respect for scientific evidence, and that the arts, including drama, can help our medical students learn to see."[34]

Embodied Practice

Increasingly, medical humanities programs are expanding to include both theater and the performing arts. In the UK, the Performing Medicine Program facilitates workshops in visual and performing arts as part of the curriculum at Barts and the London School of Medicine and Dentistry. Guest artists deliver workshops on voice, movement, improv, and acting to build confidence and develop communication and embodied presence. Exercises from Brazilian theater artist Augusto Boal's Theatre of the Oppressed are used to unearth bias and perspective. Boal used theater as a powerful political and educational tool for social change, and his exercises can be used to teach and experience myriad issues. Through the Performing Medicine workshops, artistic director Suzy Willson explains, "self-awareness can be opened up [for medical students], a space for reflection that brings with it a possibility for change and improvement."[35] In Minnesota, Hammer et al.[36] used theater in a week-long course to teach communication, empathy, and case presentation skills to students. Positive outcomes included increased confidence in presentation skills, and it was thought to be relevant at all levels.

Improvisation is commonly used to enhance communication skills, quick thinking and collaboration. In a US study on improvisation by Shochet et al., improvisation was seen to assist physicians with being able to respond to patients "in the moment" and to the need for "intuitive and improvised interpersonal responses."[37] Of the 38 respondents, 85% found the concepts highly relevant to patient care.[38] A California-based study by Hoffman, Utley, and Ciccarone used improvisation in 10 weekly workshops to teach skills thought to relate to the physician-patient relationship in place of traditional communication training with standardized patients. One respondent reported that improvisation taught them to "listen and be more human."[39] At Northwestern University, Katie Watson developed her "Medical Improv" workshops because of the similarities she perceived in these practices. She suggests that "physicians and improvisers both must develop the mental agility to think creatively and recognize patterns in rapidly changing circumstances, all while maintaining professional composure under great stress."[39] Watson notes that the goal of Medical Improv is not to produce great artists but to put students inside an artistic practice to teach them a set of skills necessary to practice their craft of medicine.[40]

Forum Theater is a method of Augusto Boal's Theatre of the Oppressed that is effective for consciousness-raising, identifying participant bias, and looking at social and political issues. In Forum Theater, audience members can stop the action of the play, step into the scene, and change the direction that the narrative of the play takes—thus ending oppression implicit in the action, changing perspective, or revealing something new. This use of direct audience involvement seeks to mitigate hierarchy and power while at the same time revealing how we are shaped and influenced by social and political determinants. A project by Kumagai et al. used Forum Theater exercises to create a faculty development workshop that facilitated "small-group discussions on potentially contentious issues involving race, gender, sexual orientation, and socioeconomic class." Findings suggested that participants found the material relevant and that in follow-up surveys the content had influenced their behavior as facilitators.[40]

Spotlight on Current Initiatives

The following section examines four different theater interventions that were implemented in Canadian programs for medical residents. The faculty involved in these initiatives all describe a strong connection to using theater as a tool to enhance reflection and self-awareness and illuminate the complexities of lived experience. Theater provides an opportunity to "get inside" another person's perspective whether through witnessing a story on the stage or performing the other. They suggested that theater can stimulate discussion of ethics, ambiguity, and complex topics that can be difficult to talk about abstractly. They felt that theater and performance practices expose residents to themes they may not feel comfortable with and provide a safer space to investigate these themes. There was a sense that this work has an impact on residents that is more profound than with standard or traditional modes of curriculum delivery. One faculty member expressed that there are very few places in which we can sit inside the ambiguity inherent in medical school and that theater allows us to do just that. Nothing has to be resolved; it can merely be a place to look more deeply, more intimately, and to learn about ourselves. Tensions inherent in the work were experienced with respect to the pressure to generate evidence that complies with quantitative and social science methods—methods that are not easily applied to theater interventions and do not always capture inherent complexity. (See chapter 10 on evaluation.)

Storytelling: Theater as Research

Paul Robert D'Alessandro, Sonia Anne Butterworth, and Gerri Frager
"Ed's Story: The Dragon Chronicles," is an example of research-informed theater where data (here in the form of interviews) are used to create a play. This verbatim play[a] was based on journal entries of a 16-year-old with advanced cancer and 25 qualitative interviews conducted after his death with his family, friends, and members of his interdisciplinary healthcare team. After phenomenological

---

a. Verbatim theatre uses the actual words of respondents as the text of the play.

analysis of Ed's journal identified major themes (adolescent development, escape from illness, changing relationships), a playwright was commissioned to create the play. "Ed's Story" generated positive responses among medical student trainees to introduce concepts of autonomy, moral distress, patient-centered care, and end-of-life care.[41] After its initial success with medical students, the use of the play was integrated into the first year Surgical Foundations Program at the University of British Columbia. With bioethics approval, 47 surgical trainees viewed a recording of the play and participated in a facilitated discussion. Trainee empathy and readiness for interprofessional learning were assessed pre- and postviewing using prospectively validated Jefferson Empathy and Readiness for Interprofessional Learning Scales. Trainees also completed confidential postviewing surveys online. Study participants were anonymous. Response rate was 54%.

A majority of residents agreed that the play was a good learning experience (65%), increased understanding of the factors that influence patient quality of life (69%), and would facilitate honest interactions with future patients (64%) and respectful interactions with other health professionals (60%). A majority of residents demonstrated an increase in empathy (56%) and readiness for interprofessional learning (57%) after viewing; however, the increased empathy score was significant only in residents with the highest pre-session scores ($p < 0.05$). The results suggest that theater-based initiatives can help residents develop competencies early in training. However, the increase in empathy scores limited to trainees with the highest preintervention scores indicates that trainees may not be brought to a standard level of competency with respect to empathy, communication, and professionalism. Thus, medical humanities educators may have to frame interventions in a way that will engage trainees more fully in learning about CanMEDS roles.

Qualitative responses indicated that residents reflected more closely upon the language they used with their patients. One trainee reflected on a palliative care consult. After watching the play, the trainee expressed guilt for being "annoyed" and wondered if he "could have been more helpful, compassionate," adding that he would be, "mindful in future, of how I choose my words." Several residents provided feedback that the play would be ideal for final-year medical students, "those who haven't seen this type of situation before," as an introduction or primer prior to the start of residency. Several felt that their real-life patient encounters in residency (ironically, the source of reflection) precluded them from maximizing learning from the session. Although they had been in residency for less than a year (and some only two months) at the time of initial viewing, the session unearthed a distinct sense of hierarchical identity amongst trainees.

Last, qualitative analysis of surgical trainee responses was mapped onto the existing Royal College Surgical Foundations curriculum. Trainee feedback demonstrated that the play addressed 10 individual competencies listed in the curriculum, including those under the CanMEDS medical expert, collaborator, professional, and communicator roles. Mapping of feedback onto existing curriculum competencies ensures that these sessions are viewed as legitimate options to deliver curriculum in interesting and enriching ways.

Suvendrini Lena is a neurologist at the Centre for Addiction and Mental Health in Toronto and a published playwright. Her play The Enchanted Loom *was professionally produced by Cahoots Theatre at the Factory Theatre in Toronto in 2016. She believes that her work as a playwright and watching the actors embody it and bring it to life has changed who she is as a doctor.*

This theater program for residents was a writing-based program in which residents read through a number of quality works from the theater cannon that concern illness as a central theme. The included plays were Peter Weiss' *The Marat Sade*, a look at life inside the Charendon Asylum during the French Revolution; Anton Chekhov's *The Seagull* and *Uncle Vanya;* Sarah Kane's *Psychosis 4.48;* Diane Flacks' *The Waiting Room;* and Margaret Edson's *Wit*. After reading the plays or excerpts from the plays, residents discussed themes and content. The residents then did their own writing for 20 to 30 minutes during which time they wrote about their own experiences in medicine. The written material was workshopped by the group, with selected material to be performed by participants. Actors or a dramaturge would sometimes join them. This collaboration was valuable as it exposed the residents to different ways of thinking. One group had a public performance of an excerpt of the material, but there was no full production of any of the work. This was articulated as an ultimate goal for participants.

Participants felt that the work allowed them to represent who they and others are and to look closely at this. They enjoyed exploring the resulting material without having to work to a specific conclusion which was felt to be "the opposite of medicine." There was consensus that using the humanities was a more effective way to teach the constructs of empathy. By grappling with both the content and the process, they were able to examine issues without the need for resolution, and this allowed enhanced understanding. Finally, in order for a program such as this to reach its full potential, both time constraints and funding are issues. It takes time for good writing to develop, and it is essential for a text to be "put on its feet" in order to bring it to life, to breathe and transform it into a live(d) experience. This requires funding for skilled artists who can work with the residents to assist them in realizing the potential of their own work. Funding is of course tied to providing evidence, which again, can be difficult to achieve through empirical models. (See chapter 11 for funding strategies.)

Performance/Improv

Dr. Jeremy Rezmovitz is a family doctor at Sunnybrook Health Sciences Centre in Toronto. He has a background in stand-up comedy and attended three months of Humber School of Comedy before leaving for more practical experience. He turned to medicine and now uses humor to teach medical residents. Dr. Lu Gao is a resident in the Department of Psychiatry at the University of Toronto.

This project was born from a research project undertaken by Drs. Rezmovitz and Gao in 2016. They compiled a literature synthesis of qualitative research on improvisation in medical education. This led them to participate in Watson's Medical Improv "train the trainer" course for health professionals at Northwestern University in Chicago. They have now successfully brought this work to the University of Toronto, where they run improv workshops for staff, students, and residents. To date they have conducted four workshops that can be applied to all levels of medical education. Their research indicated that the practice of medical improv could be connected to six out of seven of the CanMEDS roles, including professional, scholar, communicator, medical expert, collaborator, and leader, leaving out only health advocate. This robust effect is an indicator of the ways in which foundations of performance practice intersect with human interaction and provide a validation of the suitability for theater as a teaching tool in medical learning.

Improv has a set of very specific principles upon which it is based. Several of these principles can be applied to the practice of medicine. The concept of "Yes *and*" is perhaps the most foundational to improvisation. "Yes *and*" refers to the importance of saying yes to one's scene partner and adding or building onto what they have just given:

For example:

PERSON A: Hey Mom! I brought you a present.
PERSON B: I'm not your mother and you know I don't like gifts
PERSON A: Okay . . .

In this example Person B has effectively shut the scene down. He or she did not accept the offer from the scene partner and did not offer anything back. (Something that can happen all too often in the examining room.)

PERSON A: Hey Mom! I brought you a present.
PERSON B: A present! You always were very generous.
PERSON A: Surprise! I'm so generous I'm giving you my baby iguana.

In this example the scene can proceed and there are many options available because B said yes *and* took the offer and added something to it that A could then build upon. Imagine how yes *and* might influence the physician-patient relationship. It allows for curiosity and openness that can positively influence interpersonal communication.

Other principles of improv identified by participants as applicable to medical practice include listening, collaboration, and trust. Training in improvisation provides a series of exercises which are designed to build these principles into improv practice. As skills are deepened, exercises are scaffolded so that each skill can be enhanced through practice. One of the basic skills that training in improv provides is the ability to recognize and act on impulse. A return to neuroscience provides an explanation of impulse. According to Kemp, improv is a "neuronal process with words and gestures as [the] end result of these impulses."[42(p. 209)] In Dr. Rezmovitz's words: "as physicians move forward in medical education and their careers, our egos become larger and more fragile, and it can be devastating to take chances and make mistakes, whereas improv teaches us to dive in and be ready to make mistakes and learn from them." Resources that clearly define the improvisation process and include specific instructions for how to teach it include Viola Spolin's seminal *Improvisation for the Theatre*[43] and Keith Jonstone's *Impro*.[44]

Tensions uncovered in this research included lack of funding (scarce for this type of program), a focus on evidence-based outcome measures that do not capture the complexity of the work, and the skeptical perception of some residents regarding relevance to practice. While most participants' confidence improved with the workshop, some reported continued nervousness regarding presentation skills. One possible explanation for this would be that while improv is accessible and fun for participants, when there are personal blocks to taking risks in front of colleagues, a short improv course cannot deeply address them. As with many of the other programs described in this book, the greatest barriers are related to securing research grants and funding.

Performance/Embodied Practice

Dr. Skorzewska is a psychiatrist and an assistant professor at the University of Toronto Faculty of Medicine. She runs a psychiatric intensive care unit and teaches extensively using arts-based methods, in both postgraduate and continuing professional development. She started a film-craft program for psychiatric inpatients in collaboration with the Toronto International Film Festival. Dr. Skorzewska was the executive producer of an acclaimed documentary film detailing the lived experience of psychiatric inpatients called FACELESS, which has screened at festivals including Big Sky.

Medicine tends to be a cerebral practice where physicians forget that they have bodies which express things and that physical presence (or its absence) actually informs communication, collaboration, and professionalism. Little attention is paid to notions of embodiment in medical education. Dr. Skorzewska believed that a performance-based approach to body awareness would best address this. With this in mind, two of five elective arts-based sessions of three hours each were designed to encourage residents to become more aware of their bodies and the bodies of others. The sessions included a focus on how they used their voices and how they were perceived by others (based on verbal and nonverbal cues), and they were provided with the opportunity through acting exercises to gain an understanding of "what it feels like to take on the physical characteristics of others." The sessions were run by a professional actress and included basic vocal and physical acting exercises that assisted in the identification of routine habits that might convey shyness, apologizing/deference, and confidence and that could interfere with the ability to fully see and be seen. Voice exercises examined pitch, tone, intonation, and speaking style, with an intention to connect. They were taught strategies for making specific changes in how they used their bodies and voices. In addition to these hands-on sessions, there were also sessions in which the residents saw a play that contained issues central to psychiatry (though not necessarily to illness). For example, a comic play about beauty (and its effects on one's perceptions of and reactions to others) was used to challenge the residents to think about the social constructs of beauty and how they might be deeply linked to psychiatric expressions/diagnoses such as anorexia nervosa and body dysmorphic disorder. This approach was used to encourage critical thinking and awareness of individual biases that can impact real-life practice.

Theater allows the examination of complex and thought-provoking issues within a safe space. Dr. Skorzewska is most concerned with developing forms of critical thinking that can counter elements of the hidden curriculum (like unexamined power structures) and that can encourage caring, humane, and compassionate care. Because traditional medical teaching methods do not necessarily model this with any consistency, the objective of her program is "to educate residents to think critically and morally in a genuine and compassionate way and to see their patients as complex individuals."

Responses from the residents over the past five years of this elective experience have been very positive. They enjoyed this approach to learning and thinking about important yet neglected issues. They expressed that it added a dimension to how they think about their work and was a good reminder that nuance and meaning are conveyed through one's physical presence and voice. While these responses were gathered through general elective program evaluations, a more formal evaluation of the program has not yet been done. Determining the best way to evaluate their pedagogical impact has been a challenge as bio-medicine has a particular model of what constitutes evidence.

The traditional scientific model may not be best to investigate complex phenomenological and experiential learning where the learning is impacted by various factors that cannot be "controlled for" (socioeconomic status, life experience, race, gender, etc.). See her comments on these tensions in chapter 1.

Theater and medicine have commonalities where human bodies are relational sites of practice, knowledge, and complex content that can be "unpacked" and reflected upon. The possible ways to engage with theater as a learning modality are almost infinite. While most documented interventions have been done with medical students, residents can be equally impacted. In fact, it may be more beneficial to include such learning at this point in their careers when they are learning-in-action through their professional practice. Theater can take them away from the practical, rational demands of the job and provide a space in which to reflect deeply and creatively, to see and be seen, and to engage in ongoing meaning-making around human suffering and resilience.

A sample curriculum to accompany this chapter can be found online at http://cahh.ca/resources/ouplesson-plans/.

References

1. Watson K. Serious play: Teaching medical skills with improvisational theater techniques. *Art Med Educ.* 2011;86:1260–1265.
2. Hyden LC, Brockmeier J. Introduction: From the retold to the performed story. In: Brockmeier LC, Hyden J. eds. *Health, Illness and Culture: Broken Narratives.* New York: Routledge; 2008:1–15.
3. Conquergood D. Poetics, play, process, and power: The performative turn in anthropology. *Text Perform Q.* 1989;9.1:82–95.
4. Linds W. Dancing (in) the in-between. In: Schutzman M, Cohen-Cruz J, eds. *A Boal Companion; Dialogues on Theater and Cultural Politics.* New York: Routledge; 2006: 114–124.
5. Zoppi K, Epstein RM. Is communication a skill? Communication behaviors and being in relation. *Fam Med.* 2002;34.5:319–324.
6. Fallowfield L, Jenkins V, Farewell V, Sopis-Trapala I. Enduring impact of communication skills training: Results of a 12 month follow-up. *Br J Cancer.* 2003;89:1445–1449.
7. Case G, Brauer D. The doctor as performer: A proposal for change based on a performance studies paradigm. *Acad Med.* 2011;85.1:159–163.
8. de la Croix A, Rose C, Wildig E, Willson S. Arts-based learning in medical education: The students' perspective. *Med Educ.* 2011;45:1090–1100.
9. Kohn M. Performing medicine: The role of theatre in medical education. *Med Humanit.* 2011;37:3–4.
10. McCullough M. Bringing theatre into medical education. *The Lancet.* 2012;397.9815:512–513.

11. Waslenko Y. Theatre and pedagogy: Using drama in mental health nurse education. *Nurse Educ Today*. 2003;23.6:443–448.
12. Willson S. Drama for doctors. *Lancet*. 2007;369.9575:1782.
13. Boydell K. The production and disemination of knowledge: A scoping review of arts-based health research. *Forum Qual Soc Res*. 2012;13:1.
14. Wear D,Varley J. Rituals of verification: The role of simulation in developing and evaluating empathic communication. *Patient Educ Couns*. 2008;71:153–156.
15. Kohn M. Performing medicine: The role of theatre in medical education. *Med Humanit*. 2011;37:3–4.
16. Damasio A. *The Feeling of What Happens: Body and Emotion in the Making of Consciousness*. New York: Harcourt Brace; 2000.
17. Niedenthal P. Embodying emotion. *Science*. 2007; 316.5827: 1002–1005.
18. Gallese V. Mirror neurons, embodied simulation, and the neural basis of social identification. *Psychoanal Dial*. 2009;19.5:519–536.
19. Iacoboni M. Immitation, Empathy and mirror neurons. *Annu Rev of Psychol*. 2009;60:653–670.
20. Cosolino L. *The Neuroscience of Human Relationships: Attachment and the Developing Social Brain*. 2nd Kindle ed. New York: W.W. Norton; 2014.
21. McConachie B. Falsifiable theories for theatre and performance studies. *Theatre J*. 2007:59.4:553–577.
22. Levine S. *Trauma, Tragedy, Therapy: The Arts and Human Suffering*. Kindle ed. London: Jessica Kingsley; 2009.
23. Cosolino L. *The Neuroscience of Human Relationships: Attachment and the Developing Social Brain*. 2nd Kindle ed. New York: W.W. Norton; 2014.
24. Kemp, Rick. *Embodied Acting*. Abingdon, UK: Routledge; 2012.
25. Cook A. Interplay: The method and potential of a cognitive scientific approach to theatre. *Theatre J*. 2007;59.4:579–594.
26. Gray J. After the crash. *Can Theatre Rev*. 2011;146:66–88.
27. Devaney J. My leaky performances. *Can Theatre Rev*. 2011; 146:6–11.
28. Kontos PC, Mitchell GJ, Mistry B, Ballon B. Special issue: Using drama to improve person-centred dementia care. *Int J Older People Nurs*. 2010;5(2):159–168.
29. Boydell K, Jaskson S, Strauss J. Help-seeking experiences of youth in first episode psychosis: A research-based dance production.

In: *Hearing Voices* Boydell K, Ferguson B, eds. Waterloo: University of Waterloo Press; 2012; 25–44.

30. Jeffery E, Goddard J, Jeffrey D. Performance and palliative care: A drama module for medical students. *Med Humanit.* 2014;38.2:110–114.

31. Lorenz K. End of life education using the dramatic arts: The Wit educational initiative. *Acad Med.* 2004;79.5:481–486.

32. Rossiter K, Godderis R. Necessary distance: Theorizing ethnographic research–based theater. *J Contemp Ethnogr.* 2011;40:6:648–677.

33. Fetters M. The Wizard of Osler: A brief educational intervention combining film and medical reader's theatre to teach about power in medicine. *Fam Med.* 2006;38.5:323–325.

34. McCullough M. Bringing theatre into medical education. *Lancet.* 2012;397.9815:512–513.

35. Willson S. Drama for doctors. *Lancet.* 2007;369:1782.

36. Hammer R. Telling the patient's story: Using theatre training to improve case presentation skills. *Med Humanit.* 2001;37.1:18–22.

37. Shochet R, King J, Levine R, Clever S, Wright S. Thinking on my feet: An improvisation course to enhance students' confidence and responsiveness in the medical interview. *Educ Prim Care.* 2013;24:119–124.

38. Hoffman A, Utley B, Ciccarone D. Improving medical student communication skills through improvisational theatre. *Med Educ.* 2008;42:537–538.

39. Watson K. Serious play: Teaching medical skills with improvisational theater techniques. *Art and Medical Education.* 2011;86.10:1260–1265.

40. Kumagai A, White C, Ross B, et al. Use of interactive theatre for faculty developments in multi-cultural medical education. *Med Teach.* 2007;29.4:335–340.

41. D'Allesandro P, Frager G. Theatre: An innovative teaching tool integrated into core undergraduate medical curriculum. *Arts Health.* 2014;6.3:191–204.

42. Kemp R. *Embodied Acting.* Abingdon, UK: Routledge; 2012.

43. Spolin V. *Improvisation for the Theater.* Evanston, IL: Northwestern University Press; 1983.

44. Johnstone K. *Impro.* New York: Routledge; 1987.

Promoting Collaborative Competencies

Using the Arts and the Humanities to Enhance Relational Practice and Teamwork

SYLVIA LANGLOIS AND KAREN GOLD

Introduction

The arts and humanities offer important resources in developing the reflective and communicative skills necessary for patient-centered collaborative practice among health professionals. The humanities are uniquely situated to promote relational and interprofessional learning as these methods tend to be flexible, creative, and model relational authenticity.[1] Educational activities that foster empathy, mutual respect, and openness promote collaborative relationships among members of healthcare teams.[2] As the arts engage both the emotions and cognitive understanding, learners develop an appreciation of their own reactions, respect for the perspectives of others, and a deeper understanding of the experience of both team members and patients.

Although the value of incorporating the arts and humanities in undergraduate medical education has been documented, there is a paucity of literature describing the use of these methods in postgraduate training. Yet, it is at the postgraduate level where medical learners accept increasing responsibility in their area of expertise and face greater challenges when collaborating with team members and patients. The close listening and communication skills fostered by the arts and humanities enhance collaborative competencies and promote both team-building and practitioner resilience.

Interprofessional Patient-Centered Collaborative Practice

Interprofessional collaborative practice, as defined by the World Health Organization, occurs when multiple health workers from different professional backgrounds work together with patients, families, caretakers, and communities to deliver the highest quality of care.[3,4] Embedded in this concept is the notion of patient-centered care "that is respectful of and responsive to individual patient preferences, needs and values and [ensures] that . . . patient values guide all clinical decisions."[5(p. 6)] Evidence suggests interprofessional collaborative practice has a positive impact in terms of reducing the number of patient complications and length of stay, enhancing chronic disease management, improving the health of workplaces (e.g., reduced staff turnover and better relationships among team members), and reducing clinical error and mortality rates.[3,4] Collaborative practice not only has a positive impact on patient care but also contributes to practitioner well-being and resiliency, as demonstrated in the areas of medicine, surgery, and pediatrics.[6,7] Although this chapter primarily addresses the collaboration among healthcare team members, the authors recognize that patients and their family members are part of the collaborative team and that relationship with them also has an important impact on the management of the care process within the team context.

Communication problems and conflict in healthcare teams are associated with poor patient health outcomes, medical error, and even death.[8,9] Within a context of diverse patient needs and complex health systems, communication difficulties may be inevitable. Specific sources of conflict include lack of clarity regarding roles and decision-making processes, confusion over scopes of practice and accountability, as well as differences in priorities and approaches to care planning.[10] Additionally, differing communication approaches among professionals may be a contributing factor, yet within the context of close working relationships on the team, communication is critical. For example, nurses report a higher degree of workplace satisfaction when physicians address conflict with active listening rather than an authoritarian style of communication.[11] From the existing literature, we can conclude that explicitly addressing resident development of communication and collaboration competencies will contribute to enhanced team relationships and patient care.

Skills in communicating with patients and colleagues (especially close listening and empathic attunement) are foundational to effective team-based care. Empathy is generally understood as a complex skill and can be defined as "predominantly cognitive attribute that involves an understanding of patients' experiences combined with a capacity to communicate this understanding and an intention to provide help to the patient."[12(p. 287)] The notion of empathy is widely discussed with some controversy in relationship to patient care, with articles considering strategies to enhance empathy. Ironically, while studies have identified a decline in empathy throughout medical education, perception of physician's empathy is correlated with improved health outcomes and patient satisfaction.[13-16] An empathetic response can also be applied to effective team relationships, leading to "improved communication, to greater acceptance of others and by others and to attitudes that are more positive and problem-solving in nature."[17(p. 334)]

Physicians' responsibilities in promoting and leading collaboration have been clearly articulated in governing documents in North America and the United Kingdom. The issues surrounding patient-centered collaborative care are significant to residents, as they are in the process of deepening their understanding of patient care and professional roles as they navigate complex power relationships within hospital hierarchies. The General Medical Council in the United Kingdom identifies "communication, partnership and teamwork" as one of the four key learning domains.[18] In the United States, the Accreditation Council for Graduate Medical Education identifies "interpersonal and communication skills" as a core competency.[19] In Canada, the Royal College of Physicians and Surgeons competency framework for postgraduate medical education situates collaboration as a key practice domain within the Canadian Medical Education Directions for Specialists (CanMEDS) roles:

> Collaboration is essential for safe, high-quality, patient-centered care, and involves patients and their families, physicians and other colleagues in the health care professions, community partners, and health system stakeholders. Collaboration requires relationships based in trust, respect, and shared decision-making among a variety of individuals with complementary skills in multiple settings across the continuum of care. It involves sharing knowledge, perspectives, and responsibilities, and a willingness to learn together. This requires understanding the roles of others, pursuing common goals and outcomes, and managing differences.[20(p. 18)]

Relationship-Centered Practice as a Framework for Medical Care

The concept of collaborative care is closely linked to the framework of relationship-centered care. As Hovey and Craig point out, it is the "often overlooked quality of relationships between and among health care providers, patients and families that create collaborative patient-centered care."[21(p. 264)] The four underlying principles of relationship-centered practice are respect for the personhood of participants as well as their roles, acknowledgement of the role of affect in these relationships, the context of reciprocal influence, and the moral foundation of genuine relationships.[22] Healthcare practice can be conceptualized as encompassing several key relational dimensions which create a web of connectedness: practitioner to patient, practitioner to practitioner, practitioner to self, and practitioner to the broader community.[23] This conceptualization is closely aligned with Clark's framework which conceptualizes interprofessional education (IPE) and practice as encompassing three levels of relationship: relationship to oneself (professional identity), relationship to the patient (provider-patient communication), and relationship to others on the healthcare team (interprofessional teamwork).[24]

Practitioner to Patient

Considerable work has advanced the dimension of the practitioner-to-patient relationship. Much has been written about patient-centered care and its impact on health outcomes and the patient relationship. When practitioners are responsive to the needs and preferences of patients and facilitate active involvement and shared decision-making, patients express greater satisfaction with their care and report better outcomes.[14,25]

The Picker Institute, following extensive stakeholder engagement through focus groups with multiple stakeholders and a literature review, identified the characteristics of patient-centered care listed in Box 8.1.[26]

BOX 8.1 Dimensions of Patient-Centered Care

Respect for patients' values, preferences, and expressed needs
Coordination and integration of care
Information, communication, and education
Physical comfort
Emotional support and alleviation of fear and anxiety
Involvement of family and friends
Continuity of care and planning around transition
Access to high-quality healthcare

Practitioner to Practitioner

The practitioner-to-practitioner dimension of relationship-centered care is central to the concept of collaborative care. Here relationship-centered care "emphasizes that clinicians ought to listen, respect colleagues, appreciate the contributions that colleagues from other disciplines bring, promote sincere teamwork, bridge differences, and learn from and celebrate the accomplishments of their colleagues."[22(p. S6)]

Collaborative practice approaches recognize that different professions see things differently, even when they look at the same patient.[27] Seniority, medical hierarchy, and degree of experience also come into play. This is a result of professional socialization and the differences in worldviews of professions which may be more biomedical or psychosocial in focus and more disease-based or functional in nature.[24] To accommodate such differences, interprofessional teams need to create environments in which dialogue is encouraged and diverse perspectives are valued.

A relational approach to interprofessional learning and practice thus emphasizes dialogue *between/among* team members and the development of shared understandings of collaboration. Such approaches emphasize the importance of language and the implicit (and often taken for granted) meanings embedded in the language we use regarding teamwork encouraging clinicians, including residents, to explore what this term means to them within specific practice contexts.[21]

Practitioner to Self

As discussed throughout this book, the practitioner-to-self dimension emphasizes skills related to reflection and self-awareness. Self-knowledge is critical in identifying our own perspectives, values, and biases, which constitute our professional identity.[28] Informed by Schon's work on the reflective practitioner, this dimension refers to the nontechnical or aesthetic skills related to ethical discernment, value clarification, and navigating moral ambiguity.[29]

A collaborative practice lens recognizes that there are limits to one's own knowledge and validates the need for input from other professions ultimately leading to a different view of one's own professional practice and identity.[24] Medical learners may have had little opportunity to be formally introduced to concepts of mindfulness or self-reflection in their undergraduate curriculum, and these skills may be even more important as residents begin to operate at a more independent level in multidisciplinary practice settings.

Interprofessional Education to Teach Collaborative Competencies

To address the development of collaborative competencies, many pre-professional programs have implemented IPE as a foundational component to developing practice skills.[30] IPE has been defined as "members of students of two or more professions engaged in learning with, from and about each other." It is closely tied to elements of collaborative practice, which typically invites a coordinated approach to decision-making, communication and shared responsibility, accountability, cooperation, and mutual trust.[31]

Interprofessional learning spans prelicensure studies, postgraduate training, professional development (or continuing medical education), and faculty development for clinical educators. While there is debate about the exact nature of interprofessional learning outcomes, they tend to fall within three broad categories: *knowledge* of professional roles and team process, *skills* related to interprofessional communication and reflective practice, and *attitudes* of mutual respect, openness to learning, and willingness to collaborate.[32] In general, interprofessional learning activities aim to increase appreciation for the perspectives of others and cultivate a more holistic view of patient care.[24]

While the benefits of collaboration are well recognized, full collaboration is seldom practiced.[33] Despite the growing attention on these concepts, discussions on teaching and learning collaboration in health professional education have been hindered by complexity and lack of conceptual clarity. With the increasing complexity of health problems faced by healthcare practitioners in clinical practice, we have limited knowledge of the complexity of interprofessional relationships and the factors that influence collaboration, significant diversity in how collaboration is conceptualized across professions and settings, and lack of generally accepted frameworks for teaching and evaluating collaborative competencies.

Emerging literature helps identify core competencies and skills within the multifaceted concepts of teamwork and interprofessional collaboration. For example, in a large Canadian study of front-line health professionals, Suter et al. identified core competencies associated with collaborative practice.[34] They found that understanding professional roles and communicating effectively are the two most important educational competencies associated with patient-centered collaborative practice. Similarly, D'Amour et al. have tried to improve our conceptual understanding of collaboration by identifying and exploring five underlying concepts: sharing, partnership, power, interdependency, and process.[32]

Teaching and Leaning Collaboration in Postgraduate Medical Education

Teaching collaboration in postgraduate medical education is essential for preparing clinicians to practice and teach in interprofessional and team settings. In their exploration of residency as a site to gain mastery in interprofessional teamwork, Rosenthal et al. found that residents report feelings of frustration at suboptimal interprofessional relationship experiences and that team training is associated with improved resident satisfaction, less depression, and less anxiety.[35] The connection between clinician well-being and collaboration may have to do with access to mutual support and enhanced trust in day-to-day practice, improved role clarity, as well as reduced tension among team members.

We turn now to a discussion of the challenges and enablers of teaching collaboration in postgraduate medical education and through the humanities. There are a number of factors that influence the success and effectiveness of educational initiatives aimed at teaching collaboration at a postgraduate level. Some of the facilitators identified in the literature are commitment of resources from departments, coordination of diverse schedules, co-location of/ease of assembling learners, curricular mapping, the training of mentors and faculty, adequate physical space and technology, creating a sense of community and shared purpose, and positive community relationships.[31] Common themes leading to successful IPE are approaches which help learners understand their own professional identity as well as other professionals' roles on the healthcare team.[31] Learners' readiness to change is another factor that influences the effectiveness of educational initiatives aimed at improving collaboration and teamwork.[36] Additional enablers of success of IPE in postgraduate education identified in a review of the literature include stakeholder commitment, identification of champions, and a shared interprofessional vision.[37]

Oandasan and Reeves identify three areas that affect the success of interprofessional learning: factors related to the learner, the teaching environment (or approach), and the institutional environment.[38] Issues related to the learner include attitudes (i.e., resistance to IPE), professional socialization, and a culture that contributes to stereotypes, hierarchies, and lack of understanding of others. For example, they point to the "cloak of competence" (a performative stance of authority and competence not yet achieved) that medical learners feel they must develop as a contributing factor. In a study involving postgraduate learners from medicine, nursing, psychology, and pharmacy, Smith et al. discuss the role of integrated interprofessional curriculum that addresses dominant discourses within professions (i.e., misconceptions regarding roles and responsibilities, stereotypes across professions, unspoken hierarchies, and power dynamics).[39] In particular, they suggest the need for faculty role modeling of respectful relationships and open discussion of professional differences and challenges to collaboration.

Elements of collaborative practice that find their way into successful IPE experiences are responsibility, accountability, co-ordination, communication, autonomy, and mutual trust and respect as "a successful IP curriculum will ensure that students can experience, share, and practice those traits with each other."[31] Garber et al. identified attitudes toward collaboration and servant leadership (creating a community experience and shared decision-making) among residents, staff physicians, and nurses, as potentially significant variables in promoting a change in healthcare culture.[33]

Despite the conceptual complexity and "steep learning curve in forming better pedagogical constructs of how to teach IPE"[38] educational activities geared toward collaborative competencies and interprofessional teamwork have been used successfully in several residency programs. For example, internal medicine residents have been engaged in initiatives with nurse practitioner students [40,41] advanced practice nursing students,[42] chaplaincy,[43] master of public health students,[44] allied health professionals,[45] nutrition,[46] and support staff/managers.[45] The literature also describes collaborative learning with residents from family practice, psychiatry and pediatric residents and nursing staff, and clinical pharmacy and psychology students.[47–50]

Beyond positive satisfaction scores pertaining to participation in interprofessional activities, there are reports of resident learning in several dimensions. Residents identified increased knowledge of roles and responsibilities of other health professionals[40-42] and enhanced knowledge of technical skills different than their own (e.g., psychopharmacology, communication skills).[46,48] A positive change in attitudes to working with others has also been described.[49] Additionally, exposure to interprofessional learning resulted in an appreciation of the perspectives of other professionals[47] and improved confidence in working in a team-based environment.[50] Boland et al. discuss the use of an intensive immersion program for informal "side by side" team-based training of learners from family medicine, pharmacy, nursing, and psychology to improve collaborative core competencies.[50] Wagter et al. also discuss the (underutilized) role of informal daily interactions between senior physicians, residents, and nurses in clinic settings to stimulate interprofessional learning.[51] Mitchell et al. found that nurse practitioners can effectively influence attitudes and knowledge of family medicine residents through direct and indirect teaching in a clinical setting.[40]

Bandiera et al. outline the development of an interactive e-learning curriculum designed to teach teamwork and conflict resolution skills to residents.[52] (For more information see www.royalcollege.ca/rcsite/documents/canmeds/canmeds-bandiera-abner-resolution-skill-e.pdf.) Meffe et al. discuss the use of a six-part program to help learners in medicine, nursing, and midwifery using interactive educational tools (DVD scenarios, e-learning module, and role-plays) to teach the CanMEDS roles of collaborator and communicator and improve understanding of interprofessional collaboration within maternity care.[53] Research by Hanyok et al. demonstrated that didactic learning on professional roles and teamwork followed by interactions during clinic and home visits improved attitudes toward others' professional roles and enhanced respect between nurse practitioner students and internal medicine residents.[41]

Teaching Collaborative Practice with the Humanities

The relationship-centered care approach creates a structure for understanding the dynamics of collaboration. An appreciation and demonstration of the contributing elements of empathy, management of conflict, communication, and close, active listening are required to enact the relationships identified earlier, promoting both team-building, resiliency, and a patient-centered approach.

Recent research on teaching about collaboration in healthcare through the humanities illuminates key issues in curriculum development and implementation. Hall et al. hypothesized that the humanities—with their focus on "teaching us to think creatively and critically, to reason, and to ask questions"—could be infused into existing health professional curricula to meet IPE and collaborative practice goals.[54] In their article "Learning collaborative teamwork: an argument for incorporating the humanities" they discuss the development and implementation of an online learning module which addressed foundational concepts of teamwork (i.e., effective group functioning, reflective practice) and incorporated three main components: holistic care, interprofessional teamwork, and the humanities. (For more information see www.tandfonline. com/doi/abs/10.3109/13561820.2014.915513?journalCode=i jic20.)

> The humanities support a holistic and person-centered approach to care, and provide learners with new "lenses" through which to interact with clinical team members to better understand their own roles and those of others. . . . The pilot project demonstrated the difficulties and complexities of engaging students in a learning activity during busy clinical placement experiences. Although the numbers are small, the evaluation of the IECPCP&H [Interprofessional Education for Collaborative Person-Centred Practice through the Humanities] self-learning module suggests that the self-directed interprofessional module based on the humanities may valuably support IPE.[54(p. 523)]

Using a variety of care scenarios, the content was geared to learners from different professions and educational levels from prelicensure to postgraduate learners.[54] The self-directed format of the e-learning addressed the logistical and scheduling challenges of accommodating learners from different professions. The committee's experience with developing the module is discussed in more detail in Weaver's paper.[55]

Noteworthy and troubling is evidence that empathy, patient-centeredness, and an interest in interprofessional learning appear to decline throughout medical education;[14,25,31] thus addressing these attributes in residency training is critical. As demonstrated throughout this book, the arts have been used as an important resource to cultivate these attributes. Narratives, visual art, theater, and literature have been used effectively to teach empathy at various stages of medical education.[56–60] Arts and humanities have also been included in curricula to address communication, team-based collaboration, and patient-centered care.[61] Health professionals in pediatric oncology who engaged in interprofessional narrative training also reported enhanced teamwork and improved resiliency.[62] As burnout is a response to chronic emotional stressors in the workplace (characterized by cynicism and feelings of inefficacy), it is reasonable to infer that more positive interactions with others and mutual support by colleagues can mediate the negative impact of day-to-day stressors. Participating in arts and humanities activities can contribute to an acknowledgment/understanding of inherent professional differences and facilitate a move to reconciliation and expression of shared values.[54] Learning "together can break down power differentials inherent in health science disciplines/professions and can help reconcile different world-views based on shared values."[54(p. 519)] Careful planning of learning activities to develop the related competencies is essential. Key design considerations include an appreciation of the learning process, the setting of specific objectives, and engagement of creative approaches that provide the context for the use of the arts and humanities.

Key Interprofessional Teaching Principles

Learning is typically referred to as a "relatively permanent change in behavior as a result of practice or experience."[63(p. 477)] Although many learning theories can inform the use of the arts in health professional education, in this discussion we are guided by principles of constructivism and transformative learning which emphasize the learning process, the role of critical reflection in challenging assumptions and the value of social interactions in meaning-making.[64–67]

Teaching interprofessional competencies in practice settings is critical; it is in this context where residents must address the hidden curriculum that regularly challenges new concepts and approaches (see Box 8.2).

Additional consideration must be given to the level of learners asked to participate in learning activities. Since residents have increasing responsibility for dealing with the complexities of patient care, implementing activities with advanced learners from other professions may be preferable. Learning activities could also be shared with staff; however, in similar situations, residents have reported tensions when they were expected to be leaders but needed to defer to more experienced and knowledgeable staff from other professions.[47]

BOX 8.2 Strategies to Support Interprofessional Teaching in Clinical Settings[68]

Co-teaching with a colleague to model collaboration
Using the huddle concept to teach about interprofessional dynamics
Encouraging patient feedback on student learning
Reinforcing learner behaviors and correction of mistakes
Incorporating reflective activities
Seeking out faculty development opportunities
Sharing of roles and scopes of practice
Exploring power issues and establishing team culture
Assisting students to establish ground rules
Reflecting on interprofessional processes
Role-modeling interprofessional education
Assisting learners to co-create care plans with other health professionals

Interprofessional Facilitation: The Key to Fostering Collaborative Competencies

While the use of arts has implicit value in developing numerous attributes for healthcare practice, when used for the promotion of interprofessional collaboration, the application of appropriate facilitation strategies is critical. Skilled facilitators can transform multiprofessional/multidisciplinary learning opportunities (where participants work in parallel) to ones that promote interprofessionalism (where participants work collaboratively and with shared goals).

Learning with and from each other requires careful attention to group process and how participants engage with and learn from each other in order to address the goals of a task. Facilitators encourage group participants to learn and identify solutions without providing the direct answers. They guide the group process by focusing discussion and providing clarification where needed. Although they may be content experts, a group discussion does not provide a platform for the facilitator to teach.

The Interprofessional Facilitation Scale, built on a framework described by Banfield and Lackie,[69] is a valuable tool in the development of facilitation skills in an interprofessional context.[69,70] This validated scale identifies 18 items that can be used as a form of self-assessment or as a measure completed by group participants to provide feedback to a facilitator.

Conclusion

Many residents will have had exposure to the arts to some extent during their undergraduate programs, yet it is in the next phase of the medical journey where learners prepare for future practice that incorporation of art-based teaching has thus far been underutilized. Interprofessional teamwork is noted as the recommended practice model for the delivery of optimal patient care throughout North America and the United Kingdom. Collaboration is well situated in a relationship-centered model of care, with explicit focus on relationships between the practitioner and the patient, with other practitioners, and with oneself. Participation in arts and humanities learning opportunities, in addition to fostering creative problem-solving, has been shown to affect contributors of collaboration, namely empathy, close listening skills, and resilience at all levels of training. These attributes are foundational to communication, conflict management, and meaningful collaboration with team members, patients, and caregivers. Summarized case studies in this chapter provide examples of how to consider the use of humanities and art to develop collaborative competencies in postgraduate medicine. Medical residents, as well as clinicians and students from other healthcare professions, can use all of the examples provided.

A sample curriculum to accompany this chapter can be found online at http://cahh.ca/resources/ouplesson-plans/.

References

1. Konrad SC. Browning DM. Relational learning and interprofessional practice: transforming health education for the 21st century. *Work.* 2012;41(3):247–251. doi: 10.3233/WOR-2012-1295.
2. Speiser V, Speiser P. An arts approach to working with conflict. *J Human Psych.* 2007;47(3):361–366. doi: 10.1177/0022167807302185.
3. World Health Organization: Framework for Action on Interprofessional Education and Collaborative Practice. http://www.who.int/hrh/resources/framework_action/en/. Published 2010. Accessed 2016.
4. Canadian Interprofessional Health Collaborative. A National Interprofessional Competency Framework. http://www.cihc.ca/files/CIHC_IPCompetencies_Feb1210.pdf. Published February 2010. Accessed October 24, 2016.
5. Institute of Medicine. *Crossing the Quality Chasm: A New Health System for the 21st Century.* Washington, DC: National Academy Press; 2001.

6. Sulzer S, Feinstein N, Wendland C. Assessing empathy development in medical education: a systematic review. *Med Educ.* 2016;50:300–310. https://www.ncbi.nlm.nih.gov/pubmed/26896015.

7. Tsimtsiou Z, Kerasidou O, Efstathiou N, Papaharitou S, Hatzimouratidis K, Hatzichristou D. Medical students' attitudes toward patient-centred care: a longitudinal survey. *Med Educ.* 2007;41(2):146–153. https://www.ncbi.nlm.nih.gov/pubmed/17269947.

8. Kohn LT, Corrigan J, Donaldson MS. *To Err is Human: Building a Safer Health System.* Washington, DC: National Academy Press; 2000.

9. Leonard M, Graham S, Bonacum D. The human factor: the critical importance of effective teamwork and communication in providing safe care. *Qual Saf Health Care.* 2004;13(Suppl 1):85–90. doi: 10.1136/qshc.2004.010033.

10. Brown J, Lewis L, Ellis K, Stewart T, Freeman M, Kasperski J. Conflict on interprofessional primary health care teams—can it be resolved? *J Interprof Care.* 2011;25(1):4–10. doi: 10.3109/13561820.2010.497750.

11. Van Ess Coeling H, Cukr P. Communication styles that promote perceptions of collaboration, quality, and nurse satisfaction. *J Nurs Care Qual.* 2000;14:63–74. https://www.ncbi.nlm.nih.gov/pubmed/10646302.

12. Fields S, Mahan P, Tillman P, Harris J, Maxwell, Hojat M. Measuring empathy in healthcare profession students using the Jefferson Scale of Physician Empathy: Health provider-student version. *J Interprof Care.* 2011;25:287–293. doi:10.3109/13561820.2011.566648.

13. Pedersen R. Empathy development in medical education—a critical review. *Med Teach.* 2010;32:593–600.

14. Neumann M, Edelhauser F, Tauschel D, Fisher MR, Wirtz M, Woopen C, Haramati A, Scheffer C. Empathy decline and its reasons: a systematic review of studies with medical students and residents. *Acad Med.* 2011;86:996–1009. doi: 10.1097/ACM.0b013e318221e615.

15. Decety J, Fotopoulou A. Why empathy has a beneficial impact on others in medicine: unifying the theories. *Front Behav Neurosci.* 2015;8:457. doi.org/10.3389/fnbeh.2014.00457.

16. Saultz JW, Lochner J. Interpersonal continuity of care and care outcomes: a critical review. *Ann Fam Med.* 2005;3:159–166.

17. Rogers C. *On Becoming a Person: A Therapist's View of Psychotherapy.* Boston: Houghton Mifflin; 1989.

18. General Medical Council. Good Medical Practice. http://www.gmc-uk.org/guidance/good_medical_practice.asp. Published 2013. Accessed 2016.

19. Accreditation Council for Graduate Medical Education. ACGME Core Competencies. http://www.ecfmg.org/echo/acgme-core-competencies.html. Published 2003. Updated 2007. Accessed 2016.

20. Royal College of Physicians and Surgeons of Canada. CanMEDS 2015 Physician Competency Framework. http://canmeds.royalcollege.ca/en/framework. Published 2015. Accessed 2016.

21. Hovey R, Craig R. Understanding the relational aspects of learning with, from and about the other. *Nurs Phil.* 2011;12(4):262–270. doi: 10.1111/j.1466-769X.2011.00491.x.

22. Beach MC, Inui T, Relationship-Centered Care Research Network. Relationship-centered care: a constructive reframing. *J Gen Intern Med.* 2006;21(Suppl 1):S3–S8. doi: 10.1111/j.1525-1497.2006.00302.x

23. Pew-Fetzer Task Force on Advancing Psychosocial Health Education. *Health Professions Education and Relationship-Centered Care.* San Francisco, CA: Pew Health Professions Commission; 1994.

24. Clark P. Narrative in interprofessional education and practice: implications for professional identity, provider-patient communication and teamwork. *J Interprof Care.* 2014;28(1):34–39. doi: 10.3109/13561820.2013.853652.

25. Hojat M, Vergare M, Maxwell K, Brainard G, Herrine S, Isenberg G, Veloski J, Gonnella J. The devil is in the third year: a longitudinal study of erosion of empathy in medical school. *Acad Med.* 2009;84(9):1182–1191. doi: 10.1097/ACM.0b013e3181b17e55.

26. Picker Institute. Principles of Patient-Centred Care. http://cgp.pickerinstitute.org/?page_id=1319. Published 1987. Accessed October 14, 2014.

27. Clark P. What would a theory of interprofessional education look like? Some suggestions for developing a theoretical framework for teamwork training. *J Interprof Care.* 2006;20(6):577–589.

28. Kumagai A. A conceptual framework for the use of illness narratives in medical education. *Acad Med.* 2008;83(7):653–658. doi: 10.1097/ACM.0b013e3181782e17.

29. Schon D. *The Reflective Practitioner: How Professionals Think in Action.* New York: Basic Books; 1983.

30. Thibault G. Interprofessional education in the USA: current activities and future directions. *J Interprof Care.* 2012;26:440–441.

31. Bridges D, Davidson R, Soule Odegard P, Maki I, Tokowiak J. Interprofessional collaboration: three best practice models of interprofessional education. *Med Educ Online.* 2011;16. doi: 10.3402/meo.v16i0.6035.

32. D'Amour D, Oandasan I. Interprofessionality as the field of interprofessional practice and interprofessional education: an emerging concept. *J Interprof Care.* 2005;19(Suppl 1):8–20.

33. Garber J, Madigan E, Click E, Fitzpatrick J. Attitudes towards collaboration and servant leadership among nurses, physicians and residents. *J Interprof Care.* 2009;23(4):331–340. doi: 10.1080/13561820902886253.

34. Suter E, Arndt J, Arthur N, Parboosingh J, Taylor E, Deutschlander S. Role understanding and effective communication as core competencies for collaborative practice. *J Interprof Care.* 2009;23(1):41–45.

35. Rosenthal MS, Conner A, Fenick A. Pediatric residents' perspectives on relationships with other professionals during well child care. *J Interprof Care.* 2014;28(5):481–484. doi: 10.3109/13561820.2014.909796.

36. Keshmiri K, Rezai M, Mosaddegh R, Moradi K, Hafezimoghadam P, Zare MA, Tavakoli N, Cheraghi MA, Shirazi M. Effectiveness of an interprofessional education model based on the transtheoretical model of behaviour change to improve interprofessional collaboration. *J Interprof Care.* 2017;31(3):307–316. doi: 10.1080/13561820.2016.12051.

37. Lawlis T, Anson J, Greenfield D. Barriers and enablers that influence sustainable interprofessional education: a literature review. *J Interprof Care.* 2014;28(4):305–310. doi: 10.3109/13561820.2014.895977J.

38. Oandasan I, Reeves S. Key elements of interprofessional education. Factors, processes and outcomes. *J Interprof Care.* 2005;19(Suppl):39–48.

39. Smith CS, Gerrish WG, Nash M, Fisher A, Brotman A, Smith D, Student A, Green M, Donovan J, Dreffin M. Professional equipoise: getting beyond dominant discourses in an interprofessional team. *J Interprof Care*. 2015;29(6):603–609. doi: 10.3109/13561820.2015.1051216.

40. Mitchell J, Belle J, Smith C. Interprofessional education: a nurse practitioner impacts family medicine residents' smoking cessation counselling experiences. *J Interprof Care*. 2009;23(4):401–409.

41. Hanyok L, Walton-Moss B, Tanner E, Stewart, R, Becker K. Effects of a graduate-level interprofessional education program on adult nurse practitioner student and internal medicine resident physician attitudes towards interprofessional care. *J Interprof Care*. 2013;27(6):526–528.

42. Kowitlawakul Y, Ignacio J, Lahiri M, Khoo SM Zhou W, Soon D. Exploring new healthcare professionals' roles through interprofessional education. *J Interprof Care*. 2014;28(3):267–269. doi.org/10.3109/13561820.2013.872089.

43. Hemming P, Teague P, Crowe T, Levine R. Chaplains on the medical team: a qualitative analysis of an interprofessional curriculum for internal medicine residents and chaplain interns. *J Relig Health*. 2016;55(2):560–571.

44. Gupte G, Noronha G, Horny M, Sloan K, Suen W. Together we learn: analyzing the interprofessional internal medicine residents' and master of public health students' quality improvement education experience. *Am J Med Qual*. 2016;31(6):509–519.

45. Curran V, Heath O, Kearney A, Button P. Evaluation of an interprofessional collaboration workshop for post-graduate residents, nursing and allied health professionals. *J Interprof Care*. 2010;24(3):315–318.

46. Lawrence J, Knol L, Clem J, Tucker M, Henson C Higginbotham J, Strieffer R. Perceptions of team performance and professional stereotypes in interprofessional education among nutrition students, medical students, and medical residents. *J Acad Nut Diet*. 2016;116(9):A89.

47. Van Shaik S, Plant J, O'Brien B. Challenges of interprofessional team training: a qualitative analysis of residents' perceptions. *Educ for Health*. 2015;28(1):52–57.

48. Wilkening G, Gannon J, Ross C, Brenna J, Fabian T, Marcsisin M, Benedict N. Evaluation of branched-narrative virtual patients for

interprofessional education of psychiatry residents. *Acad Psych.* 2017;41:71–75. doi:10.1007/s40596-016-0531-1.

49. Baker C, Pulling C, McGraw R, Damon J, Dagnone D, Hopkins-Rosseel D, Medves J. Simulation in interprofessional education for patient-centred collaborative care. *J Adv Nurs.* 2008;64(4):372–379.

50. Boland DH, Scott MA, Kim H, White T, Adams E. Interprofessional education collaborative competencies in side-by-side training of family medicine, nursing, and counselling psychology trainees. *J Interprof Care.* 2016;30(6):739–746. doi: 10.1080/13561820.2016.1227963.

51. Wagter JM, van de Bunt G, Honing M, Eckenhausen M, Scherpbier A. Informal interprofessional learning: visualizing the clinical workplace. *J Interprof Care.* 2012;26(3):173–182. doi: 10.3109/13561820.2012.656773.

52. Bandiera G, Hawryluck L, Abner E, Glover Takahashi S, Richardson D. Teaching conflict resolution skills through a curriculum web initiative. International Conference on Residency Education—What Works. Abstract 208. Royal College of Physicians and Surgeons of Canada. 2009. http://www.royalcollege.ca/rcsite/documents/canmeds/canmeds-bandiera-abner-resolution-skille.pdf. Accessed May 2, 2017.

53. Meffe F, Moravac C, Caccia N. An interprofessional education/collaboration (IPE/C) program in maternity care: development, implementation, evaluation and adaptability. International Conference on Residency Education—What Works. Abstract 152. Royal College of Physicians and Surgeons. http://www.royalcollege.ca/rcsite/documents/canmeds/canmeds-meffe-maternity-care-e.pdf. Published 2010. Accessed May 2, 2017.

54. Hall P, Brajman S, Weaver L, Grassau P, Varpio L. Learning collaborative teamwork: an argument for incorporating the humanities. *J Interprof Care.* 2014;28(6):519–525. doi: 10.3109/13561820.2014.915513.

55. Weaver L, McMurtry A, Conkin J, Brajtman S, Hall P. Harnessing complexity science for interprofessional education development—a case example. *J Res Interprof Pract Educ.* 2011;2(1):110–120.

56. Charon R. *Narrative Medicine: Honoring the Stories of Illness.* Oxford: Oxford University Press; 2008.

57. Wikstrom BM. A picture of a work of art as an empathy teaching strategy in nurse education complementary to theoretical

knowledge. *J Profess Nursing.* 2003;19(1):49–54. doi: 10.1053./
jpnu.2003.5.

58. Dow A, Leong D, Anderson A, Wenzel R, VCU Theater-
medicine team: using theater to teach clinical empathy: a pilot
study. *J Gen Intern Med.* 2007;22(8):1114–1118. doi: 10.1007/
s11606-007-0224-2.

59. Shapiro J, Morrison E, Boker J. Teaching empathy to first year
medical students: evaluation of an elective literature and medicine course. *Educ Health.* 2004;17(1):73–84. doi: 10.1080/
13576280310001656196.

60. Shapiro J, Duke A, Boker J, Ahearn CS. Just a spoonful of
humanities makes the medicine go down: introducing literature
into a family medicine clerkship. *Med Educ.* 2005;39:605–612.
https://www.ncbi.nlm.nih.gov/pubmed/15910437.

61. Acai A, McQueen S, McKinnon V Sonnadara R. Using art for
the development of teamwork and communication skills among
health professionals: a literature review. *Arts Health.* 2017;1:60–
72. doi.org/10.1080/17533015.2016.1182565.

62. Sands S, Stanley P, Charon R. Pediatric narrative oncology:
interprofessional training to promote empathy, build teams, and
prevent burnout. *J Support Oncol.* 2008;6:307–312. https://www.
ncbi.nlm.nih.gov/pubmed/18847073.

63. Lachman S. Learning is a process: toward an improved defini-
tion of learning. *J Psych.* 1997;131:477–480. http://dx.doi.org/
10.1080/00223989709603535.

64. Hean S, Craddock D, O'Halloran, C. Learning theories and
interprofessional education: a user's guide. *Learn Health Soc Care.*
2009;8(4):250–262. doi: 10.1111/j.1473-6861.2009.00227.x.

65. Vygotsky LS. *Mind in Society: The Development of Higher
Psychological Processes.* Cambridge, MA: Harvard University
Press; 1998.

66. Mezirow JE. Perspective transformation. *Adult Educ. Q.*
1978;28:100–110.

67. Mezirow, JE. *Fostering Critical Reflection in Adulthood: A Guide
to Transformative and Emancipatory Learning.* San Francisco, CA:
Jossey-Bass; 1990.

68. Lie D, Forest C, Kysh L, Sinclair, L. Interprofessional education and practice guide no. 5: interprofessional teaching for
prequalification students in clinical settings. *J Interprof Care.*
2016;30(3):324–330. doi:10.3109/13561820.2016.1141752.

69. Sargeant J, Hill T, Breau L. Development and testing of a scale to assess interprofessional education (IPE) facilitation skills. *J Contin Educ Health Prof.* 2010;30(2):126–131. doi: 10.1002/chp.20069.
70. Banfield V, Lackie K. Performance-based competencies for culturally responsive interprofessional collaborative practice. *J Interprof Care.* 2009;23(6):611–620. doi: 10.3109/13561820902921654.

Teaching History of Medicine/ Healthcare in Residency

EDWARD SHORTER AND SUSAN E. BÉLANGER

Introduction

This chapter is intended to give clinicians who intend to teach the history of medicine to residents a bit of context. So it is not just about current models for doing this kind of teaching but also about how the field of medical history has evolved. Even though the main focus is residents, we write about undergraduate instruction as well, for it is here that lessons have been learned and approaches sharpened. Where does this field of medical history come from? What is its usefulness in the larger context of medical humanities, and what does one actually teach?

The notion of teaching the history of medicine to specialist trainees is feasible only if specialties themselves exist. While teaching medical history to undergraduates is age old, teaching residents is rather new. (Readers interested in the history of medical education might consult the works of Kenneth M. Ludmerer, most recently *Let Me Heal: The Opportunity to Preserve Excellence in American Medicine.*[1]) As recently as the last quarter of the nineteenth century, the idea of specialist training was virtually unknown except in disciplines such as psychiatry that required specialized facilities. In the UK, for example, clinicians saw themselves as generalists and regarded specialism as overly narrow for the broadly educated gentleman or -woman.[2] Joel D Howell wrote in 2016, apropos Ludmerer's *Let Me Heal*, "Since around the turn of the twentieth century, the organization of medical care has increasingly relied on categorizing physicians as members of specific specialties."[3] So, while specialist trainees would be interested in the history of their specialty, there was not necessarily an official specialty whose history one could isolate.

The development of the specialties as an historical event in medicine is, in itself, an interesting development and dovetails with the explosion of medical developments that took place in the 20th century. In teaching residents, it is therefore important to convey a sense of the excitement of studying history, as well as of the possible clinical and professional benefits that a good knowledge of history might bring. This chapter explains some of the benefits, but we would be happy if residents and their teachers come away from this section of their medical humanities curriculum enthusiastic about past triumphs and tragedies of their field and resolved to do better. Also, some of these books are jolly good reads!

Theoretical Discussion of the Role of the History of Medicine in the Undergraduate and Postgraduate Medical Curriculum: Past Traditions

It would be overly grand to claim that there is a "theory" of the role that history might play in the postgraduate curriculum. Historians tend to be practical people. Yet over the years certain insights have formed about the usefulness of history in the training of postgraduate physicians.

One camp sees history as an *anchor for civic values*. Medical training was once full of talk about values and community leadership; here, historical images played a role. As Charles K. Clarke said in 1919, as a six-year curriculum was about to be introduced, "The changes made in the curriculum will enable students to acquire a broader culture. . . . Six years may seem a long time to remain at College, but those who have acquaintance with the history of medicine are fully convinced that it is not possible to graduate a cultured and practical physician in less time."[4] At some universities, it was once common for the undergraduate curriculum to include courses on French, anthropology, and history. Not that curriculum planners thought that a knowledge of French or anthropology would be useful in the practice of medicine but that the medical students, scarce out of high school, would better step into later roles as community leaders if they knew something other than anatomy and physiology. This was an era when physicians were seen as the backbone of a kind of community elite, and this kind of leadership role demanded a broader educational background.

This concept of civics training greatly weakened after the Second World War as physicians played less and less of a role as community leaders and medical schools began demanding that applicants acquire intellectual diversity during their *previous* undergraduate training in arts and science, rather than the medical faculty itself offering this kind of education. For some time, the stipulation of a broad undergraduate background virtually vanished from undergraduate medical admissions requirements, although this trend is now reversing.

As for postgraduate training in medicine, the focus has always been on acquiring the knowledge base necessary for specialist practice rather than on civics training. As humanities topics were eliminated from medical education programs, bioethics stepped in to take their place. Yet bioethics, drawing together as it does law and philosophy, is not the same thing. In any event, the purpose of medical training at any level is no longer seen as forming community leaders, and the entire philosophy of civics training was really limited to the first half of the 20th century.

To the extent that some medical schools encouraged humanistic training in their postgraduate programs, it was in the form of a year-long rotation at the great medical schools of the UK and the Continent: London, Paris, Berlin, and Vienna. Here, the medical graduates might acquire a second language; certainly there were benefits from exposure to the leading minds of the day, which were to be found in the European capitals and not in Bethesda, Maryland (where the National Institutes of Health would flourish after the Second World War). American and Canadian residents and postgraduate fellows returned from these journeys with a firmer understanding of the history of medicine and with a new cosmopolitanism. Clarence B. Farrar, for example, later professor of psychiatry in Toronto, prided himself on his knowledge of the German he had acquired during a year's residency at Heidelberg with the histopathologist Franz Nissl and with Emil Kraepelin, the founder of modern psychiatric nosology.[5] Other clinicians returned home with similar experiences. Whether this made their relations with their patients more humane is unclear.[6]

A second approach sees knowledge of medical history as an *anchor of wisdom*. This orientation commenced in the hands of such clinician-scholars as Heinrich Ludwig von Attenhofer in Vienna, who began lecturing on medical history in 1808.[7]

At the undergraduate level, "medical history" (*Medizingeschichte*) was once a required course, hated by the students and included on the exam. Here the underlying philosophy was medicine as a storied source of learning that had built upon the wisdom of the ages. It was not unusual, at one point, for medical schools to demand from their graduates a reading knowledge of Latin. And the heart of *Medizingeschichte* was often learning the Greek and Latin roots of medical terminology.

At the postgraduate level in Europe, the medical doctoral dissertation (called habitationes—obligatory at the time) was to review the previous literature on the subject going back to the Ancients. This is a far cry from the brief review of recent contributions expected today in scientific papers. And postgraduate students writing "habilitations," a big book following the doctoral dissertation, which qualified one for teaching, were expected to have a comprehensive grasp of the previous history of the subject. Here, the view was that the past represented a vast storehouse of useful knowledge, not civics training or ethical preparation, and that learned scholarship must be, essentially, historical in nature.

This view has not been entirely abandoned in graduate training on the Continent, yet it has been starkly modified. Essential to the grasp of one's subject became an understanding of its biochemistry, later of its molecular biology; what hoary figures who lived a hundred years ago might have thought about the issue in question remains today largely uninteresting. From the viewpoint of medicine as a science, one can scarcely quibble with this approach. From the viewpoint of medicine as a humanistic combination of the art and science of practice, this rather mechanistic approach to the past does not fit readily into the medical humanities concept.

The third approach is the history of medicine as an *anchor of humanistic learning and practice*. Within medical education there has been a general reaction to the notion of postgraduate training as mills producing practitioners who may be technically superb in their specialties but who, in human relations and moral values, seem to verge on obtuseness. Part of the concept of medical humanities means softening the science of medicine with something of the art of medicine, and it is from historical models that we learn that the art of medicine was once a living reality.

The art of medicine was once valued, not because practitioners believed that medicine was necessarily unscientific but because it added a psychological dimension to doctor-patient relations;[8] a human relationship of this intensity could not possibly be sustained on the basis alone of an understanding of biochemistry or molecular biology. Patients, in this view of postgraduate medical education, are seen as partners in a relationship, and they have emotional needs. It is the duty of the competent practitioner to fulfill, to the extent possible, some of these needs and expectations. And it is the role of the history of medicine to offer past models of this two-way communication.

This tradition of medical education as a repository of humanistic learning goes back to the turn of the century. In 1910 Will Mayo, one of the founders of the Rochester clinic named after his family, said, in the words of historian W. Bruce Fye, "Doctors must think of each patient as a whole person despite progressive specialization."[9] In the 1930s a formal "patient as a person" movement evolved, associated with William R. Houston (1936)[10] and George Canby Robinson (1939).[11] Both Houston and Robinson offered sage, historically founded advice about psychological elements in the doctor-patient relationship, particularly in the treatment of symptoms without lesions, later referred to as somatization, or "psychosomatic illness." These doctors may be seen as founding figures in medical humanities, as they had great respect for the psychological lessons that might be learned from the past. (Robinson, the more influential of the two, merited a long entry in the *Dictionary of American Medical Biography*.[12])

Robinson urged greater engagement with "the social and emotional aspects of illness . . . [but] freed from emotional reactions in the doctor. Feelings such as pity need not be suppressed or disregarded, but they must become a motive rather than an emotion." Here Robinson cited the mid-19th-century Scottish physician John Brown, who wrote the moving story in *Rab and His Friends* (1859) about what he, Brown, had learned studying medicine at Minto House Hospital. It was that emotions, such as loyalty, can interfere with care. "The tenets of science can be applied to investigation in this field, and in fact unless they are applied, not much of permanent value is likely to emerge." Harkening back to the generalist physicians of the past, Robinson urged the creation of a new sort of " 'general physician' who combines in part the attitudes and methods of the internist, the psychiatrist, the hygienist and the medical social worker." Such a physician, Robinson explained, would "know his patients as total individuals and can treat and guide their health through struggles with social adversity and social incapacity, relieve their psychogenic symptoms, and give them adequate medical care for illness or injury that does not require hospitalization."[13] Robinson's biographer Theodore Brown adds, "Creation of this new specialist, like teamwork between hospital-based internists and medical social workers, would thus patch up the existing system of medical care."[14] Here, the lesson of history is that medicine once knew well how to care for psychosomatic illness but then lost the thread.

Recent Developments in Europe and the United States

Joining medical humanities has been challenging for recent proponents of medical history. "Infiltrating "historical content into medical-school curricula offers no guarantee of continued success.[15] What is the problem here? Poorly articulated arguments, uninterest, or hostility among medical educators and health science students? Yes and no, recent scholarship has concluded: Despite their frustration with their marginal position in medical education, the striking continuity of historians' arguments for the discipline—and their ability to engage at least some members of the health professions and general public—shows s stability "that is a real accomplishment in a field as obsessed with novelty as medicine."[16]

Recent Developments in Europe

The rigorous systematizing of the classical tradition has not been entirely abandoned in European medical education. In some centers, the former classical model has been supplanted by departments or institutes dedicated to the medical and health humanities (such as those established in Switzerland at the Université de Genève[17] and Berlin's Charité university medical center[18]), which integrate the study of history with other disciplines including anthropology, bioethics, and literary or cultural studies.

In 1993 the General Medical Council of the UK, in a report *Tomorrow's Doctors*, recommended that medical history be included in a new program of interdisciplinary studies.[19] Following this recommendation, in 1996 Liverpool University introduced a compulsory history of medicine component into the medical curriculum, and in the UK medical history began to gain wide acceptance, often in connection with nearby units of the Wellcome Institute for the History of Medicine. In this spirit of medical humanities, one scholar noted, "The study of the history of medicine can remind students of the transient nature of much medical knowledge and of the importance of keeping up to date with developments."[20] In many centers, medical history and bioethics have been merged into a single program. Although this will be seen as a plus for medical humanities, it is not necessarily a ringing endorsement of the benefits as such of studying the past.

The Johns Hopkins Approach

Following the 1873 will of Baltimore merchant Johns Hopkins, a hospital named after the benefactor was opened in 1889, teaching only graduate students; in 1893 an undergraduate medical school followed. The Hopkins medical institutions quickly became the leading North American medical faculty and were firmly based on scientific learning and laboratory investigation.

In teaching medical history to residents, the model offered by Johns Hopkins has been exemplary, combining a native North American enthusiasm with the deep learning of the Continent. Here, several threads came together. Hopkins combined an emphasis on the basic sciences and laboratory investigation (imported from France and especially Germany) with close clinical instruction by full-time professors; furthermore, it entailed a deep respect for wide-ranging learning and interests in the humanities (especially history and literature); finally, it incorporated a humanistic approach to education and practice. Johns Hopkins insisted, for example, on a knowledge of French and German among its incoming medical students,[21] and William Osler, who arrived at Johns Hopkins University Hospital in 1889 as physician-in-chief, personified the caring bedside manner—as well as a particular interest in the history of medicine. In the mid-1890s, he founded the Johns Hopkins Medical Historical Club.[22]

It was Henry Sigerist who implanted the tradition at Johns Hopkins of teaching medical history. Sigerist was born in Paris in 1891, trained in medicine at Zurich and Munich, and, as a pupil of the great Karl Sudhoff in Leipzig, he abandoned clinical medicine and became a professor of the history of medicine, first at Leipzig then, after 1932, at Johns Hopkins. Sigerist directed the Institute of the History of Medicine at Johns Hopkins, founded in 1929, and made it into an important seedbed of US medically trained medical historians.[23]

The Hopkins model of the 1890s differed sharply from the trade-school approach previously in effect at most North American medical schools. Before the "Flexner Report" of 1910, which insisted that basic science underlie medical training, American medical education *grosso modo* had been modeled on a kind of "apprentice-ship" system where, after two years of classroom instruction, one basically learned by doing. One entered medicine directly after high-school graduation and had little scientific understanding of what was, essentially, a craft. No role for history here (also, post-graduate training was minimal to nonexistent). So the Hopkins model opened the door to a modern, science-based residency and created a role for the history of medicine in understanding one's place in this new world. Thus, far from being antihistorical, scien-tific training in medicine was, essentially, "prohistorical."

These efforts at Johns Hopkins bore fruit. By 1951, according to Wilhelm Moll, a survey of the American Association for the History of Medicine demonstrated that 37 of the 79 schools med-ical schools had regular history of medicine courses. There were five departments or full-time chairs of the history of medicine.[24]

From the History of Medicine to "Health Humanities"

The concept of "health humanities" was adumbrated in 1947 in the journal *Isis* by the great Dutch historian of science George Sarton who founded the journal. He wrote, "The new historians of science . . . will be the best coordinators of scientific education in all its forms, and what is even more important they will con-stitute the necessary links between our technical barbarians and the well-meaning humanists . . . humanizing the men of science and the engineers and reminding them always of the traditions without which our lives, however 'efficient,' remain ugly and meaningless."[25] As Sarton intended, "medical humanities" became the more inclusive term. The aim was that, to engage with other health professionals, medical historians should try to integrate their own offerings into wider curricula and training programs. There is, however, a danger that solid historical content may degenerate into pablum when asked to "integrate" into other disciplines. Teaching the historical "background" of salient bioethical questions is not the same as teaching history. As we have seen from the previous discussion, there are good reasons for offering the history of medicine as a free-standing subject and not as ancillary to some other program. In 1956 psychiatrist Ilza Veith described "The function and place of the history of medicine in medical education." She considered the history of medicine "indispensable in a well-rounded medical curriculum" and anticipated her studies of "hysteria" (which would become a well-known later book) that showed how important it was to have historical perspective on a diagnosis of this nature.[26]

On Teaching the History of Medicine to Undergraduates and Residents Today

The history of medicine as a medical humanity thus has a pedigree. What is the case today? In 2000, Barron H Lerner, an internist and medical historian at Columbia University College of Physicians & Surgeons, suggested various ways of making the history of medicine relevant to medical students and trainees, such as emphasizing medicine as a "profoundly social enterprise," evident in the history of forced sterilization, chronic fatigue syndrome, and Lyme disease. "Many institutions," he added, "are also beginning to use the rubric of 'medical humanities' to formally explore the patient's experience of illness. Medical history should be integral to any such curriculum."[27] In a major review article published in 2015 ("Making the Case for History in Medical Education"), four leaders in the field argued vigorously for the inclusion of history in North American medical curricula.[28] In a January 2017 feature by the New York University Medical Humanities website ("Why History of Medicine?"), Lerner continued to emphasize the importance of history as "a key subject within the medical humanities" with many valuable lessons for "modern health professionals." "History reminds us," he said, "that medicine has been—and always will be—a social process. That is, even as we learn more about the molecular and genetic basis of disease, and use increasingly sophisticated statistical methods to evaluate our interventions, this knowledge does not provide 'objective' truths. Rather, those who generate such scientific information do so within a complicated cultural and political setting."[29]

Teaching medical history to undergraduates and postgraduates thus emerges as a new reality. In 2012, a survey of anesthesia departments in the United States established that 54% of the programs that responded to a questionnaire reported that they "had at least one faculty member with an interest in history of anesthesia, and 45 percent of programs included lectures related to history of anesthesia in their didactic curriculum."[30]

As for the teaching format, a variety of approaches to undergraduate education have been reported over the past three decades, many of them recommending more engaging formats than the traditional lecture. During the late 1980s, two professors at Michigan State University designed and successfully implemented a case study ("focal-problem") course based on John Snow's investigation of the 1854 cholera outbreak in London. [31] George Rosen at Columbia University, who was probably the dean of American medical historians, in 1956 dilated upon the teaching of the subject to undergraduates, especially from the viewpoint of social history. [32] One should not overlook a more recent discussion of teaching medical history to undergraduates using case studies.[33]

Librarians at Northwestern University in 2012 provided a useful model for inserting medical history into the curriculum by introducing students to rare books and special collections.[34] (The online appendix, "Guidelines for Reviewing Primary Literature," provides some highly practical and academically sound tips for health professions trainees and others venturing into this specialized field.[35])

Also, in 2012 a team from Louisiana State's Health Sciences Library described a database-searching course for third-year medical students that incorporates insights into medical history using the *Edwin Smith Surgical Papyrus*, a digitized ancient text.[36] As for anesthesia, in 2014, two members of the Department of Anesthesiology at the University of Massachusetts Medical School at Worcester described use of novels, movies, and site visits as "alternative methods" in teaching the history of the discipline.[37] In 2016 two scholars at the University of Minnesota described their work in teaching medical history through the use of primary sources,[38] including oral histories,[39] material culture, and special collections.[40]

Resources integrating medical history with medical humanities exist as well. One of the four main sections of Thomas Cole et al.'s *Medical Humanities: An Introduction* covers "history and medicine" and includes, among other topics, "The Doctor-Patient Relationship," "Educating Doctors," and "The Health of Populations."[41] It was the late Roy Porter who penned the magisterial *The Greatest Benefit to Mankind: A Medical History of Humanity from Antiquity to the Present*.[42] Jacalyn Duffin has offered an authoritative account in *History of Medicine: A Scandalously Short Introduction*.[43] And Edward Shorter's *Doctors and Their Patients: A Social History*[44], while not a comprehensive history of medicine, is nonetheless a useful guide to the vicissitudes of the doctor-patient relationship.

Exemplary Works

It is important that residents be exposed to the best that medical history has to offer, and, in one sense, herein lies its interdisciplinarity: Medical history is more than a retirement pastime for old doctors but is rather a vibrant interdisciplinary field of active scholarship. As we have seen, the history of medicine began life in Europe and reached a kind of apex with the works of Karl Sudhoff and Henry Sigerist. What has propelled it into the 21st century, however, is the arrival in the 1960s of PhD social historians who are, generally speaking, not medically trained but who see medical history as an entry portal to larger societal questions such as the history of gender, the history of concepts such as intimacy, and the history of "the body," giving concreteness to this otherwise rather ephemeral notion.

To illustrate: In 2014, Shauna Devine wrote a model history of the role of the Civil War in the rise of modern surgery.[45] The history of eugenics and genetics has been fertile ground, and Pauline M.H. Mazumdar's classic *Eugenics, Human Genetics and Human Failings* (1992) has spawned a series of studies.[46] Thomas Laqueur at the University of California has pioneered the "history of the body" concept with works on the cultural construction of sex and on the history of masturbation.[47] We learn from this scholarship that even the most intimate events in the body's long temporal arc are somehow socially constructed. (While we highlight PhD scholarship, it cannot be denied that some knowledge of medicine is important even for PhDs: Mazumdar and Duffin are also MDs, Edward Shorter took the two-year basic medical science program at a major medical school, and Thomas Laqueur participated in a clinical rotation in gastroenterology.)

The history of psychiatry has not fallen short, given the obvious appeal to social historians of psychiatry. Ben Shephard, who wrote the standard work on "shell shock," actually started out as a journalist.[48] Paul Lerner broke the mold on "hysteria" as a female concept by writing *Hysterical Men: War, Psychiatry, and the Politics of Trauma in Germany*.[49] And Hannah S Decker brought a historian's skills to the history of psychiatry's diagnostic guide, the *Diagnostic and Statistical Manual of Mental Disorders,* especially the third edition in 1980, known as DSM-III.[50] Key works in the history of psychiatry might include Edward Shorter, *A History of Psychiatry*.[51] In the library of every serious scholar of psychiatric history should be Richard Hunter and Ida Macalpine's magnificent *Three Hundred Years of Psychiatry*,[52] an edited compilation of essential primary texts. Readers will also find helpful Hugh Freeman's edited volume, *A Century of Psychiatry*.[53]

In teaching residents, these titles serve as valuable illustrations of the excitement and scholarly excellence in the field of medical history. This is but a small sample of a huge range of high-quality scholarship from the pens of social historians, few of whom have medical training. The history of medicine is thus genuinely inter-disciplinary, drawing alike from medicine and history; conveying this to residents is an important teaching objective, if only because medicine itself is "interdisciplinary," in a sense, and the clinical gaze must be widened to include the patient's social background.

A sample curriculum to accompany this chapter can be found online at http://cahh.ca/resources/ouplesson-plans/.

References

1. Ludmerer K. *Let Me Heal: The Opportunity to Preserve Excellence in American Medicine*. New York: Oxford University Press, 2015. See also Ludmerer, *Learning to Heal: The Development of Medical Education*. New York: Basic Books, 1985; and Ludmerer, *Time to Heal: American Medical Education from the Turn of the Century to the Era of Managed Care*. New York: Oxford University, Press, 2005.
2. See Stevens R, Medical practice, in Walton J, et al., eds., *The Oxford Companion to Medicine*. Oxford: Oxford University Press, 1986, I, 755–769. On the lack of differentiation in British medical practice around 1900 see James Crichton-Browne's various memoirs, including *The Doctor's After Thoughts*. London: Benn, 1932.
3. Howell JD. A history of medical residency. *Rev Am His*. 2016; 44: 126–131.
4. Shorter E. *Partnership for Excellence: Medicine at the University of Toronto and Academic Hospitals*. Toronto: University of Toronto Press, 2013, 651–652.

5. See Shorter ECB. Farrar: A life, in Shorter ECB, ed., *TPH: History and Memories of the Toronto Psychiatric Hospital, 1925–1966*, Toronto: Wall & Emerson, 1996, 59–96.

6. See on this Bonner TN. *American Doctors and German Universities*. Lincoln: University of Nebraska Press, 1963.

7. Lesky E. *Die Wiener Medizinische Schule im 19. Jahrhundert*. Graz: Böhlau, 1965, 618.

8. Shorter E. *Doctors and Their Patients: A Social History*, new ed. New Brunswick, NJ: Transaction, 1993.

9. Fye WB. The origins and evolution of the Mayo Clinic from 1864 to 1939: A Minnesota family practice becomes an international "medical mecca." *Bull Hist Med*. 2010. 84: 323–357, 336.

10. Houston WR. *The Art of Treatment*. New York: Macmillan, 1936.

11. Robinson GC. *The Patient as a Person*. New York: Commonwealth Fund, 1939.

12. Kaufman M, et al., eds. *Dictionary of American Medical Biography*. Westport, CT: Greenwood Press, 1984, II, 643–644.

13. Robinson, *Patient as a Person*, 400, 410.

14. Brown TM. George Canby Robinson and "The Patient as a Person," in Lawrence C, Weisz G, eds., *Greater Than the Parts: Holism in Biomedicine, 1920–1950*. New York: Oxford University Press, 1998, 135–160, 151; Robinson quotes from Brown.

15. Duffin, J. Infiltrating the curriculum: An integrative approach to history for medical students, *J Med Humanit*. 1995; 16 (3): 155–174. In a subsequent issue she teams up with a bioethicist to teach an interprofessional class. Weisberg M, Duffin J. Evoking the moral imagination: Using stories to teach ethics and professionalism to nursing, medical, and law students. *J Med Humanit*. 1995; 16 (4): 247–263. Fuller J, Olszewski [Cocks] MM. Medical history in Canadian undergraduate medical education, 1939–2012. *Can Bull Hist Med*. 2013; 30 (2): 199–209.

16. Jones DS, Greene JA, Duffin J, Warner JH. Making the case for history in medical education. *J Hist Med Allied Sci*. 2015; 70(4): 623–652.

17. Louis-Courvoisier M, Wenger A. How to make the most of history and literature in the teaching of medical humanities: The experience of the University of Geneva. *Med Humanit*. 2005; 31: 51–54.

18. Kiessling C, Mueller T, Becker-Witt C, Bergenau J, Prinz V, Schleiermacher S. A medical humanities special study module on

principles of medical theory and practice at the Charité, Humboldt University, Berlin, Germany. *Acad Med.* 2003; 78(10): 1031–1035.

19. General Medical Council. *Tomorrow's Doctors.* London: Author, 1993.
20. Macnaughton J. The humanities in medical education: Context, outcomes and structures. *Med Humanit.* 2000; 26(1): 23–30. http://dx.doi.org/10.1136/mh.26.1.23
21. Flexner A. *Medical Education in the United States.* New York: Carnegie Foundation, 1910, 234.
22. Bliss M. *William Osler: A Life in Medicine.* Toronto: University of Toronto Press, 1999, 249.
23. See Brown TM, Foo E. Sigerist HE. Medical historian and social visionary. *Am J Public Health.* 2003; 93(1): 80.
24. Moll W. A brief survey of the teaching of the history of medicine in the United States. *Bull Hist Med.* 1962; 50: 207–213.
25. Sarton G. Preface to Volume 37: Qualifications of teachers of the history of science. *Isis* 1947. 37: 5–6.
26. Veith I. The function and place of the history of medicine in medical education, *J Med Educ.* 1956; 31(5): 303–309. Veith, *Hysteria: The History of a Disease.* Chicago: University of Chicago Press, 1965.
27. Lerner BH. From laennec to lobotomy: Teaching medical history at academic medical centers. *Am J Med Sci.* 2000; 319: 279–284.
28. Jones DS, Greene JA, Duffin J, Warner JH. Making the case for history in medical education. *J Hist Med Allied Sci.* 2015; 70(4): 623–652.
29. Lerner B. Why history of medicine? New York University, Division of Medical Humanities, http://www.med.nyu.edu/medicine/medhumanities. Accessed January 23, 2017.
30. Desai MS, et al. The teaching of anesthesia history in US residency programs: Results of a nationwide survey. *J Clin Anesthesia.* 2012; 24: 101–103.
31. Brody H, Vinten-Johansen P. Teaching the history of medicine by case study and small group discussion. *J Med Humanit.* 1991; 12(1): 19–24.
32. Rosen G. An orientation course in the history of medicine. *J Med Educ.* 1956; 31, 680–683.
33. Brody H, Vinten-Johansen P. Teaching the history of medicine by case study and small group discussion. *J Med Humanit.* 1991; 12(1): 19–24.

34. Shedlock J, Sims RH, Kubilius RK. Promoting and teaching the history of medicine in a medical school curriculum. *J Med Libr Assoc.* 2012; 100(2):138–141.

35. Shedlock J, Sims RH, Kubilius RK. Guidelines for reviewing primary literature. *J Med Libr Assoc.* http://dx.doi.org/10.3163/1536-5050.100.2.014. 222112.

36. Timm DF, Jones D, Woodson D, Cyrus JW. Combining history of medicine and library instruction: An innovative approach to teaching database searching to medical students. *Med Ref Serv Q.* 2012; 31(3): 258–266.

37. Desai MS. Desai SP. Alternate methods of teaching history of anesthesia. *Anesth Analg.* 2014; 118: 438–447.

38. Tobell DA. Teaching medical history with primary sources. *Bull Hist Med.* 2016; 90(1): 124–127.

39. Tobell DA. Teaching with oral histories. *Bull Hist Med.* 2016; 90(1): 128–135.

40. Hendrickson L. Teaching with artifacts and special collections. *Bull Hist Med.* 2016; 90(1): 136–140.

41. Cole T, et al. *Medical Humanities: An Introduction* New York: Cambridge University Press, 2015.

42. Porter R. *The Greatest Benefit to Mankind: A Medical History of Humanity from Antiquity to the Present.* London: HarperCollins, 1997.

43. Duffin J. *History of Medicine: A Scandalously Short Introduction,* 2nd ed. Toronto: University of Toronto Press, 2010.

44. Shorter E. *Doctors and Their Patients: A Social History,* new ed. New Brunswick, NJ: Transaction, 1993.

45. Devine S. *Learning from the Wounded: The Civil War and the Rise of American Medical Science.* Chapel Hill: University of North Carolina Press, 2014.

46. Mazumdar PMH. *Eugenics, Human Genetics and Human Failings: The Eugenics Society, Its Sources and its Critics in Britain.* London: Routledge, 1992.

47. Laqueur T. *Making Sex: Body and Gender from the Greeks to Freud.* Cambridge: Harvard University Press, 1990; Laqueur, *Solitary Sex: A Cultural History of Masturbation.* New York: Zone Books, 2003.

48. Shephard B. *A War of Nerves: Soldiers and Psychiatrists in the Twentieth Century.* Cambridge: Harvard University Press, 2001.

49. Lerner P. *Hysterical Men: War, Psychiatry, and the Politics of Trauma in Germany, 1890–1930.* Ithaca: Cornell University Press, 2003.

50. Decker HS. *The Making of DSM-III: A Diagnostic Manual's Conquest of American Psychiatry*. New York: Oxford University Press, 2013.
51. Shorter E. *A History of Psychiatry*. New York: Wiley, 1997.
52. Hunter R, Macalpine I. *Three Hundred Years of Psychiatry*. London: Oxford University Press, 1963.
53. Freeman H, ed. *A Century of Psychiatry*, 2 vols. London: Mosby-Wolfe, 1999.

Difficult Conversations

Evaluating the Medical Humanities

MARTINA KELLY

[T]he striving for certainty, a feature of western intellectual
thought since the times of Plato and Aristotle, has come to an
end. There is no one right answer to a situation, no formula of
best practices to follow in every situation, no assurance that
any particular act or practice will yield the results we desire.[1]

Introduction

Evaluating medical humanities (MH) is an ongoing conversation between science and art. On one side, seeking scientific credibility, medical education builds ivory towers of outcomes and objectives, single best answer questions, and standardized, objective examinations. Here, everything is measurable, ideally using a validated or Likert-type scale. The chief concern of tower dwellers is how educational interventions cause quantifiable changes, such as in knowledge, skills, or opinion. Below these towers, arts and humanities sprawl outward, as a slum. Diverse and curious, slum residents view learning outcomes with suspicion as forms of social control. They question everything and gauge impact qualitatively through music, language, or the body. The concern here is not with quantitatively measurable impact but with far more subtle and personal shifts in subscription to values or gains in tolerance and appreciation. The dwellers of the slum world of qualitative studies look up to the ivory towers of medical science.

Those of us promoting the MH need to learn how to bridge these opposing worldviews. Nietzsche,[2] in the *Birth of Tragedy*, spoke of two opposing aesthetic worlds of art, the Apollonian and the Dionysian. In this chapter, I draw playfully on these ideas, to make an analogy between Apollonian and Dionysian approaches to evaluation of the MH. Within this chapter, MH is defined as application of techniques of reporting, interpreting, and theorizing developed by the traditional humanities fields to phenomena within the medical field.[3] In the opening section, I briefly review some arguments regarding the value of MH in medical education, proceeding then to my primary purpose of providing some initial guidance to colleagues interested in MH teaching on how to evaluate a small educational project. In doing so, I draw on some examples from the literature. Due to the paucity of research on MH in postgraduate settings, many examples are situated in undergraduate programs, but the principles are transferable to the postgraduate setting. Throughout, I draw on my experience as a doctor, teacher, and medical education researcher.

Evaluation is the "systematic collection and analysis of information related to the design, implementation, and outcomes of a program, for the purpose of monitoring and improving the quality and effectiveness of the program."[4] Evaluation means making a value judgement about information or activities. Recognizing different values lies at the heart of the hostilities sometimes expressed toward the topic of evaluation of the MH. This was well demonstrated in the discussion that followed publication of a review on MH,[5] which focused on outcomes, and subsequent commentaries which questioned a narrow focus on endpoint rather than process.[6,7] These arguments were not just methodological, quantitative over qualitative; rather they were axiological. Axiology is the science of how we "value values." Just as in clinical practice we learn to respect each other's values, having a healthy awareness of traditional medical (Apollonian) and humanities (Dionysian) values is just as helpful when it comes to evaluating or researching the MH.

Let's start with some Greek mythology: Apollo was the god of music, the sun, truth, and healing. An Apollonian view is dominated by rational, logical thought, built on analysis of the conscious mind, with an objective, knowable truth as a reachable endpoint. This represents the biomedical perspective traditionally dominant in medical education, where teaching and learning are presented as linear, logical, consequential, and computational. In contrast, Dionysus was the god of wine, fertility, and theater. A Dionysian view values intuition and imagination and prioritizes unconscious modes of experience, where subjective truth is conveyed through representational symbols. This mirrors the potential of MH to develop innovative, interpretative ways of experiencing the clinical messiness of daily practice, explore emotional responses, and promote subjectivity as a legitimate response to clinical uncertainty. What is of particular relevance to the MH community is that good art, in the Hellenic tradition, does not value Apollonian or Dionysian views over each other but emphasizes the generation of new ideas by creating tension between them. While scientific medicine offers a primarily Apollonian view, we have opportunities to exploit the eclectic multidisciplinary Dionysian nature of MH and to develop novel evaluation approaches out of the tension of this coincidence of opposites.

Before looking at the question of how to do this, it is pertinent to review some of the debates regarding evaluation that permeate the existing MH literature. For many of us, introducing a novel course on MH is born out of personal interest and passion. As educational leaders, we have great opportunities to open our learners to new ways of experiencing medicine. Beware, though, of Pandora's Box! MH is serious business, yet with little agreement on what it is or how it should be taught.[8,9] We can risk in our naive enthusiasm stumbling into potentially heated discussions with our arts and humanities colleagues, who with their own critical lenses question not which Canadian Medical Education Directions for Specialists (CanMEDs) competence we shall evaluate but *if* MH should be evaluated at all.[6,7]

In this introductory section, I have stressed that evaluation is not necessarily a measure (the outcomes of science) but an articulation of the quality of an act of learning as expressed by its relative value. This questions a "one-size-fits-all" evaluation process, as learners may experience differing value outcomes for a common element of learning.

The Value Proposition of Medical Humanities: Homeostasis or Productive Instability?

What is the value of MH in medical education? In many programs, the role of MH is instrumental or ornamental.[10–12] Instrumental functions of the MH relate to how study of MH helps physicians in their day-to-day work, for example use of visual arts to improve observation skills or use of narratives to improve empathy. In an ornamental role, students are encouraged to study MH as a means of coping with the stress of a career in medicine, often reflected in feedback such as "relaxing." Here, the MH are palatable and pleasurable, offering enrichment to counter empathic decline and tailored to the goals and priorities in the practice of medicine.

Use of humanities, where art is used to maintain a state of "homeostasis,"[8] co-opted to promote a utilitarian view of Western values is of grave concern to a number of leading MH scholars.[6,13–15] Rather, they argue that a fundamental role of MH is to be provocative and critical, where students should be encouraged to question the structures and systems within which they learn. By challenging our taken-for-granted assumptions, a key role for MH is to create a type of educational "productive instability" as in the dynamism of a complex, adaptive system—so perhaps we should not be surprised when students perceive MH as a countercultural activity.[16,17] Evans[13] distinguishes between government–like, externally imposed, mandatory regulation, potentially represented by science-based forms of evaluation, and governance—a collective, autonomous, self-regulatory processes, arguing that the former is incompatible with the values of MH. He advocates the need for governance, where through a process of authentic partnership and assimilation, novel standards of practice can emerge.

The different ways we value MH are reflected in the choices we make as educators, reflected in our learning aims, objectives, and outcomes (should we choose to use them); our choice of course material; and the role of assessment and course evaluation. Bleakley[8] sees value in introducing students to more avant-garde art and humanities to question ingrained pieties and conservative values in medicine and sees value in art meeting medicine in the clinic, rather than students being hived off to museums and galleries. After all, there are strong parallels between the "white cube" of the gallery and the "white cube" of the clinic. Belling[18] notes a tendency to prioritize certain poets over others and a preference for small, impactful pieces of writing for medical education purposes. Dennhardt et al.[19] conducted a scoping review on MH teaching in medical education and emphasized the relationship between what a course is aiming to achieve and how evaluation is approached. The research team provided a useful framework linking the focus of teaching with research and evaluation methodologies. Dennhardt and colleagues suggested that MH teaching takes place on a continuum, art as expertise (which focuses on skill building), art as dialogue (which promotes perspective taking and focuses on relationships), and art as expression or transformation (art for personal growth and activism). In turn, these different functions of MH can be investigated by different methodologies, where skill-building courses are more suitable to examination using traditional scientific modes of evaluation and the dialogical role of the arts is better investigated using more qualitative approaches, ranging from interpretative to more critical approaches (see Table 10.1).

It is important to note here that art can be used to teach social activism, social critique, and social justice, areas of concern becoming increasingly important to medicine that has, historically, claimed to be apolitical.

Having reflected on what you actually want to achieve with your medical teaching, it is time to get started. What follows are some practical tips to consider as you go along. I start with some general guidance. I then provide some examples of evaluation models, starting with traditional scientific (Apollonian)

TABLE 10.1 Framework Linking Teaching Focus, Methodology, and Methods in Medical Humanities

	Art as Expertise (skills)	Art as Dialogue (perspective-taking, relational)	Art as Expression (art for personal growth)	Art as Transformation (art for activism)
Teaching Focus	Art as Expertise (skills)	Art as Dialogue (perspective-taking, relational)	Art as Expression (art for personal growth)	Art as Transformation (art for activism)
Purpose	Explain, predict, control, cause-effect	Understand, interpret, reconstruct		Critique, transform, emancipate
Methodology	Traditional Experimental/ Quasi-experimental	Qualitative (e.g., grounded theory, phenomenology, narrative analysis)		Critical theory Discourse analysis Institutional ethnography
Method	Randomized trial Pre–post test design	Interviews, focus groups, observation, field notes, researcher reflexivity		

Note. Based on framework from Dennhardt et al.[19]

Methodology refers to the beliefs regarding knowledge, usually based on the theories and philosophies that guide the research process. Methods refer to the tools, techniques, or procedures used to gather data.

models, before giving some examples from qualitative research (Dionysian). For each, I highlight some of the strengths and weaknesses of approaches to highlight the tensions between them. Finally, with a sense of mischief, I introduce readers to Hermes, the rascally son of Apollo, famous for his mixed messages, by introducing readers to more novel forms of arts-based research (ABR).

Getting Started: Scope and Standards

What's the plan? Introducing a new course or seminar is exciting, and there is often lots of energy at the outset. Ironing out initial content, learning goals, and delivery can result in evaluation as an afterthought when the course is finished. But, like any teaching endeavor, preparation is key—there is nothing worse than realizing you did not collect baseline data or get appropriate ethical permission ahead of time, if, for example, you want to do a before/after intervention study. A useful exercise is to write a formal protocol—think ahead about who, what, where, when, and how. Plan for contingencies—what do you do if you have more or fewer participants than you anticipated? Discuss the protocol with colleagues and solicit feedback ahead of time, so that you can adjust your plans as needed.

Whose opinion matters? A key question is "Who is the evaluation for?" Are you carrying out an evaluation to justify the course to the dean? Writing up the course as part of a teaching portfolio or sharing new insights with an international audience?[20] Thinking about your intended audience will help determine the scope of the project.

Evaluation, scholarship, or research? Evaluation often draws on research methodologies—but not every evaluation is a research project.[21] The focus of evaluation is on change, often for local use with practical application—what actions can be taken as a consequence of the evaluation to improve a specific offering? Research, in contrast, explores broader questions, situated within a theoretical framework with a view to generating new understandings. While there is overlap between evaluation and research, the scope of questions asked and the standards used to judge their quality are significantly different.[22] Balmer et al.[22] give an example of how these issues become problematic, when it comes to examining free-text comments from program evaluations. Evaluation standards will focus on how useful the feedback is and how feasible it is to act upon the feedback and assumes that they are representative of stakeholder perspectives. Research standards, in contrast, will question issues of transferability—for example to other programs—and how credible and dependable the data are. Familiarize yourself with the criteria by which your work will be judged, be it evaluation,[20] educational scholarship,[23,24] or, say, qualitative research,[25-27] ideally as part of your planning strategy.

What's been done before? Reading colleagues' experiences, examining the methods used, the lessons they learned, and their ideas for future research can inform your evaluation. This is particularly important in MH because of the elective nature of many residency program initiatives, small sample size, and frequent criticisms of MH evaluations. Find a study you admire, dealing with content you value or answering questions similar to your own. It may be possible to collaborate with colleagues working in an area or to replicate their study.[28] Possibilities for networking and further training in MH are described in chapter 1 and in the appendix.

A particular challenge searching for humanities work is that much material, especially by humanities scholars, is unlikely to be indexed in PubMed—books and book chapters are the preferred publishing medium for many humanities researchers. Additionally, much humanities research is likely to use qualitative modes of inquiry, catalogued using a wide range of terms. For this reason, working with a librarian is invaluable to develop your search strategy. Some initial resources to help extend your literature search are given in Table 10.2.

TABLE 10.2 Sample Resources for Literature Searching

Resources to Identify Medical Humanities Material	Advantage
Scopus Google Scholar (especially advanced function)	Indexes journals in virtually every discipline
ProQuest Dissertations	Searches for theses, a valuable resource in the humanities
Google Books	Identifies relevant chapters within books, often missed by conventional library search systems
OpenGrey http://www.opengrey.eu/ Duke University Medical Centre Guide to Searching the Grey Literature http://guides.mclibrary.duke.edu/c.php?g=158169&p=1035967	Searches for grey literature—literature that is not formally published in journals or books.[29] It includes government reports, conference proceedings, and unpublished clinical trials
http://www.gold-foundation.org/programs/research/mtl/	The Gold Foundation funds systematic reviews on humanism which are listed on its homepage
Resources on how to identify medical humanities material	
Material written by Andrew Booth[30] http://methods.cochrane.org/qi/welcome	Andrew Booth, University of Sheffield, UK has written extensively on search strategies for qualitative research. He is co-convenor of the Cochrane Collaboration's Qualitative and Implementation Methods Group. The website is a useful resource for anyone interested in undertaking a qualitative synthesis.
Wilczynski, Marks, Haynes[31]	Tips for finding qualitative studies in CINAHL
Walters, Wilczynskil, Haynes[32]	Tips for finding qualitative studies in EMBASE

An additional starting point is to read existing reviews of MH.[5,12,19,29-34] The reference lists of these articles can direct readers to more specific studies for a given topic or arts-based method. These reviews and related commentaries[6,7,35] also reflect some of the ongoing controversies or critiques that will help you anticipate issues in your evaluation approach. Bleakley[8] has a chapter (chapter 9) devoted to "Evaluating the Impact of Medical Humanities Provision" in which he problematizes the quasi-scientific approaches of "measuring impact" to consider how we might grapple with issues such as individual response and values clarification and education. For example, Bleakley considers tolerance of ambiguity an outcome of MH interventions.

While most readers are likely familiar with quantitative reviews, a novel suite of review methods collectively termed qualitative evidence synthesis (QES) have recently been used to synthesize findings from qualitative studies and are well suited to MH. QES is defined as "any methodology whereby study findings are systematically interpreted through a series of expert judgments to represent the meaning of the collected work."[36] QES reviews are increasingly recognized as contributing to healthcare decisions as recognized by Cochrane Collaboration,[37] the US Agency for Healthcare Research and Quality, and the UK National Institute for Heath and Clinical Excellence. However, they are relatively novel to medical education, and their diverse methodologies and terminologies, such as meta-ethnography, meta-narrative review, and realist review, can be confusing. A basic overview of QES is provided at http://www.goldfoundation.org/programs/research/mtl/introduction-qualitative-evidence-synthesis/.[38] Given the prevalence of qualitative research within MH, QES is a potentially exciting means to review MH initiatives. Two prime examples of QES reviews in MH have been recently published.[19,29] QES reviews require the same attention to searching, quality appraisal, and synthesis as quantitative reviews, and interested readers are encouraged to work with an experienced health librarian and colleague with expertise in qualitative research, preferably QES itself.

Rigorous evaluation requires time. It benefits also from shared expertise. Working with residents and students can be helpful, but can you offer them the level of support they need, being respectful of their time demands? Collaboration with colleagues who have methodological expertise is beneficial, so interdisciplinary approaches are favored in medical education scholarship—both for publication and funding. Failing that, you need to budget for expert help. For example, if using a questionnaire, do you need to do a power calculation to estimate sample size or access statistical advice on analyzing the results, particularly the validity of using the specific questionnaire in your population? If considering qualitative work, do you have a budget for transcription costs, and do you need digital recorders or software to help with analysis? What is your timeline? Will you need ethics approval? Ethical standards for evaluation and research differ according to institutional policies (at the hospital and university levels). Similar to preparing a protocol, detailing a budget including protected research time can help scope the project out—ahead of time.

Be realistic. Perhaps one of the biggest pitfalls is over-reach. Keep it simple! There is a lot of rhetoric about how MH promotes empathy, tolerance for ambiguity, and moral development. These are multifaceted constructs, often poorly defined within the medical education literature. The complexity of medical education as a whole makes isolating certain attributes difficult, perhaps impossible. Rich, in-depth case studies can provide interesting insights and, if well executed, can extend understandings well beyond the local context.[39-41]

Study Design: Evaluation in Evolution

Familiar forms of evaluation in medical education are outcomes-focused, using experimental or quasi-experimental design. There is a growing skepticism that these traditional, linear Apollonian approaches can capture the Dionysian messiness of medical education, especially at the postgraduate level. Teaching and learning are not always as predictable as we might assume. Learners come with different levels of experience; what is taught in one school may not transfer well to another; and education is constantly subject to external factors, be it accreditation policies or funding issues. This has led to an interest in studying education as a system—where the sum is greater than the parts. Systems theory and complexity theory are increasingly used in educational program evaluation, as they can appreciate and accommodate the uncertainty and dynamic change inherent in many educational initiatives and allow them to adapt to shifting contexts.[42-44] The focus of these approaches is that they extend our understanding of outcomes to include outputs and impact. They also specifically include examinations of process.

Since MH evaluations are commonly condemned due to shortcomings in "proving" outcomes, process evaluation constitutes an important extra dimension. While MH is often criticized for its "fuzzy, fluffy nature," the growing awareness of the value of moving beyond metrics to include soft intelligence is influential in healthcare policy.[45] Here, soft intelligence includes not only information (data) but the *processes and behaviors* associated with application of insights and use of local knowledge (narrative, explanatory, and particular). After all, "fuzzy logic" (degrees of truth rather than absolutes) is now commonly accepted in science thinking.

Experimental/Quasi-Experimental Evaluation

This approach is probably the most intuitive for clinically trained educators who regard randomized controlled trials the gold standard and believe it is possible to isolate certain elements of a course and examine them. Common examples of this approach to evaluation include *intact-group design* and *time-series experiments*.

In the intact-group design learners are randomly assigned to one of two groups, one of which is exposed to the traditional program and the other to the newer program. In a time-series study, learners are observed before and after the program, which is most useful when immediate and long-lasting changes in behavior or knowledge are anticipated.

A number of such studies are reported in the MH literature, particularly in the domain of visual arts.[46-48] In a study at Yale, 146 first-year medical students were randomly allocated to receive instruction via lecture, which reviewed radiographic images or a fine art intervention in which they studied paintings in detail. The course was evaluated using a pre- and posttest, which consisted of grading learner observations of dermatology photographs. Posttest scores were significantly higher for the fine art intervention group.[48] A similar study using a cluster design, controlled trial, where groups of family physicians and primary care nurses were randomly allocated to control or intervention group, is reported by Kirklin et al.[49] These types of studies lend themselves well to evaluation of postgraduate observation skills. The limitation of such studies is that, while an objective judgement is made about skill acquisition, there is no indication that values have changed. A first-year resident might be able to better observe the details of a radiology image, but does he or she still objectify the patient?

A smaller study, comprising 32 students, evaluated 90-minute art rounds, used visual thinking strategies as its intervention, and evaluated outcomes using standardized scales such as the Communication Skills Attitudes Scale[50] and a variation of Budner's Tolerance of Ambiguity scale.[51,52] The authors demonstrated a significant increase in tolerance for ambiguity and positive views toward healthcare professional communication skills.[53] Again, while a shift might be made in a scale score, how does the person act in an ambiguous clinical context, such as discussing a borderline key test result with a patient? MH education promises to increase both visual acumen and empathy.

BOX 10.1 Questionnaires Often Used in Medical Humanities Studies

Jefferson Scale of Physician Empathy[56,57]
Communication Skills Attitudes Scale[50]
Tolerance of Ambiguity Scale[51,52]
Patient-Practitioner Orientation Scale[58,59]

Although the use of quasi-experimental designs is popular, and there have been calls for more of them in MH,[12] there are drawbacks. The medical educational environment does not typically afford the rigorous controlled conditions necessary for this type of design, so internal validity is low. For example, many MH courses remain elective, especially in the residency context, which presents challenges for randomization. Graham et al.[54] measured empathy before and after an elective humanities module and found an improvement of pre–post scores but concluded it was difficult to know if this was a result of the educational intervention or a propensity for empathic students to choose a humanities elective.[54] Ethical considerations and resources may not facilitate the running of two similar courses, one of which prevents learners from participating in a potentially useful learning exercise. Additional considerations relate to sample size and statistical power—this is particularly important when thinking about using a standardized questionnaire (Box 10.1) and its suitability within your specific educational context. Do not forget to check for copyright permission when using a standardized questionnaire. If you are considering designing your own questionnaire, some useful tips are given by Artino et al.[55]

Kirkpatrick's Four-Level Evaluation Model

Kirkpatrick,[56] a British industrialist, devised a model of evaluation used in medical education. He proposed four "levels" of evaluation, outlined in Table 10.3.

TABLE 10.3 Kirkpatrick's Levels of Evaluation

	Kirkpatrick Level	*Measured By*
1	Learner satisfaction	Likert scales Narrative comments
2	Learning as a result of the program	Assessment data Knowledge—written (e.g., essays) Skill demonstration (e.g., OSCE)
3	Change in learner behavior	Simulated encounters Observation in the clinical setting
4	Results in the large context	Improved patient care, team performance, or health savings

Kirkpatrick's model is popular because it is simple. Researchers commonly use Likert scales measuring stakeholder satisfaction and the results of student assessments to evaluate programs. But these have shortcomings. Satisfaction is a poor surrogate for educational effectiveness, and—as Cook reminds us—assessment focuses on learners whereas evaluation should focus on programs.[20,57] Recently, the Kirkpatrick model has come under scrutiny.[58,59] As originally described, the model represents a hierarchy of outcomes, where "a" leads to "b" in a sequential manner. This is supposedly independent of process and pays no attention to unanticipated outcomes. This emphasis on outcome rather than process pays little attention to confounding variables. Levels 3 and 4 are difficult to measure and may not always be appropriate in education.[59,20] Cook[60] warns of the danger of adopting patient outcomes as the holy grail of medical education, citing small sample sizes, potentially biased outcome selection, teaching to the test, and the difficulty of establishing a causal link as dangers. In particular, linking what a physician does to patient outcomes is problematic as it fails to account for patient preferences, healthcare system factors, and the impact of other healthcare providers and family members. In other words, the effect of education becomes diluted by a multitude of unpredictable factors.

In response to these criticisms, Kirkpatrick's children proposed a New World Kirkpatrick Model, emphasizing that levels are not predictive. They did, however, retain a focus on predefined outcomes identified early in the planning process.[61]

From Outcomes to Process

Following Dennhardt's model[19] (see Table 10.1), educators who move further away from measuring objective outcomes or skills make greater use of qualitative and mixed methods research to evaluate MH courses. They usually gather qualitative data from interviews, focus groups, or observation. Mixed methods, as the name suggests, includes quantitative and qualitative data[62] in order to evaluate both process and outcomes.

Because qualitative data collection and analysis is rarely taught at undergraduate level, it is wise to ask for help. Many universities have qualitative researchers, some with specialist interests in medical education. Setting up a meeting to get some advice and direction ahead of a project is time well spent. Contact your postgraduate medical education office for links to colleagues doing this work.

Qualitative inquiry is often synonymous with thematic analysis, but there are a number of different types of qualitative methodologies, each of which has its own theoretical and philosophical roots. It is these theoretical orientations that gives different methodologies their unique flavors. Good qualitative research makes effective use of theory to frame the research question, determine methods, and inform the results. The range of "-ologies" can be overwhelming and is like learning a new language. A brief overview of some approaches commonly used is given in Table 10.4.

If a resident is considering qualitative research, it would be beneficial to start the project with a research elective to hone the research question and explore options with some experienced colleagues. This creates an opportunity for some upfront reading, while simultaneously starting a literature review and ethics

TABLE 10.4 Some Exemplar Qualitative Methodologies

Qualitative Methodology	Father Discipline	Features
Grounded theory	Sociology	GT is one of the most widely used qualitative methodologies in medical education. The approach originated from the work of sociologists Glaser and Strauss[63] and has evolved over time. Contemporary medical education is often "constructivist" GT[64] to reflect the interpretative nature of data collection and analysis, whereby knowledge is actively constructed and co-created by researchers and participants.
		The intent of GT is to develop theory, "grounded" in the data. Common features of GT research are iterative data collection and analysis, theoretical sampling, line by line coding, and use of constant comparison.
Ethnography	Anthropology	The aim of ethnography is to describe, analyze, and interpret cultural beliefs and practices. Key features of ethnography are close observation in a natural setting, interviews with participants in that setting, and document review.[65]
		Institutional ethnography is a form of ethnography which specifically looks at how people interact within a given context, to show how these relationships become institutionalized.[66]

(continued)

TABLE 10.4 Continued

Qualitative Methodology	Father Discipline	Features
Phenomenology	Philosophy	Phenomenology is not a single "method" per se but approaches are influenced by the thinking of different philosophers such as Husserl, Heidegger, Gadamer, and Ricoeur. Using this approach, researchers attempt to understand a phenomenon, often by exploring the lived experience of participants. The role of the researcher as an interpretative instrument is a particular feature of phenomenological research, as is attention to language.[67,68]
Narrative analysis	Literary criticism	Narrative analysis finds its roots in literary criticism and, in education, is influenced by the work of John Dewey.[69] Researchers adopting this approach consider our lives as "storied"; people use story to interpret their experiences and make them personally meaningful. Narrative inquiry is the study of experience as story. Stories are told, retold, and relived in storied ways. Stories are told to another person—in this way, narrative inquiry is relational,the researcher interprets the story, based on his or her own personal story. Common devices in narrative analysis are attention to time, place, and person.

TABLE 10.4 Continued

Qualitative Methodology	Father Discipline	Features
		For example, when does the story start (past/present tense); where is the story set, what details are given (and which are absent), who are the characters in the story, how do they relate to each other?[70-72]
Discourse analysis[73-75]	Sociology and linguistics	Discourse is a family of research methodologies which stem from Marxist social theory, ethnomethodology, and linguistics. Their common assumption is that spoken words represent and influence social action. "Macrolinguistic" discourse research is typically orientated toward the work of Michel Foucault. It examines large bodies of textual material to explore how language structures society. At the other extreme, "microlinguistic" discourse research examines fine-grained features of spoken or written language to examine how social structure and action are constructed linguistically.[73] "Mesolinguistic" analysis (actually, combined macro- and microlinguistic analysis) examines the interplay between structuring effects of language, writ large, and human agency as represented in finer linguistic detail.[74]

Note: GT = grounded theory.

application. Creswell[63] and Patton[64] are core texts on qualitative research. Additional starter references are provided in the appendix. As qualitative research can generate large volumes of textual data, it is useful to pilot some initial data collection and analysis prior to committing to a full-scale research project.

Two Examples of Qualitative Studies in Medical Humanities

Two studies, which evaluated use of narrative in medicine, are provided by Arntfield[17] and Kumagai.[86–89]

In a study to explore the perceived influences of narrative medicine training on the CanMED competencies of communication, collaboration, and professionalism, Arntfield[17] (the author of chapter 2) used a mix of open-ended surveys at baseline and 1½ years after the course, supported by a focus group. The researchers examined data using grounded theory.[90] While participants reported that narrative was important and effective in supporting them to explore non-expert competencies, they also reflected on the misconceptions about narrative medicine and barriers to its adoption within the wider culture of the school. What is nice about this study is its attention to detail: by richly describing the context and using rigorous theoretically based methodology, the authors were able to develop a conceptual model which extended their findings beyond their own institution to help other educators using narrative approaches.

Kumagai,[86,87,89] the author of the foreword for this book, has examined the value of stories through a series of studies based on a mandatory two-year preclinical program in which students meet patients with a chronic illness and reflect on their experiences. In the first study, focus groups were used to describe what students learned about living with chronic illness.[86] In a later study, individual interviews were chosen to more fully explore how students understood interacting with patients with diabetes.[89] Again, using grounded theory, Kumagai and colleagues devised a narrative theoretical scheme to understand whether this promoted a patient-centered approach to patient care. Kumagai then reflected on his experiences to propose a conceptual framework for the use of illness narratives, grounded in theories of empathy and moral development, promoted through pedagogical strategies which promote the value of "making strange."[87,91] Apart from rich descriptions of the data, a strength of Kumagai's work is that it is theoretically embedded. His thoughtful approach to a single program has evolved over time, which these studies show. While not typical program evaluation per se, his work shows how deep engagement with pedagogy and theory can contribute to a wider promotion of humanities within medical education and offset the common criticism of qualitative research, which is its lack of generalizability. It is a good model of process-based reflection as evaluation, again with drawing out value as its main concern rather than number crunching.

Combining Outcome and Process: The Logic Model and the Context, Input, Process, Product Model

The logic and the context, input, process, product (CIPP) models provide specific styles of evaluation that combine attention to outcomes and process. Both find their roots in systems theory. The logic model[92] pays attention to the relationship between program components (Table 10.5) and context by mapping the resources and the sequence of events, connecting the need for a program with its results. An example of the logic model is described in a framework for evaluating arts for health and well-being by Public Health England.[93]

A more complex approach to integrating outcome and process in program evaluation is provided by the CIPP model (Table 10.6).[94] The CIPP approach consists of four sets of studies, which can be integrated or conducted independently. The advantage

TABLE 10.5 The Logic Model

Activity	Innovations or Changes Planned
Output	Tangible things produced
Outcome	Changes in "behavior, skills, status and level of functioning" of participants
Impact	Changes in organizations, communities, or systems.

of the CIPP model is that it allows for both articulation and appreciation of the complex dynamic, nonlinear relationships that characterize many educational initiatives. This type of approach requires careful planning and is probably more suited for larger pieces of curricular work.

Revolution: Art *as* Evaluation

> Writing about music is like dancing about architecture.
>
> –ANONYMOUS

So far, we have reviewed modes of evaluation commonly employed in medical education. Yet what about evaluating the humanities in their own terms and in ways intrinsic to each discipline? After all, even the nonliterary scientist knows that literature is critically approached through a variety of modes of exegesis of texts. Despite consistent cries for innovative forms of evaluation for the MH,[7,18] it is somewhat surprising that greater use has not been made of ABR in MH. "Arts-based research" is an umbrella term used to describe a range of research activities such as storytelling, poetry, music, dance, theater, and the visual arts. ABR is most established in education[74-76] but is increasingly being used in health research.[31] Playing Hermes, god of mischief, I briefly introduce readers to ABR, where experience—of and for itself—constitutes evidence.[77]

TABLE 10.6 The Context, Input, Process, Product Model

	Context	Input	Process	Product
Aim	Identifies and defines goals and priorities. Assesses needs, problems, assets, opportunities	Explains why and how a given approach was selected and explores alternative options. Considers resource implications and looks at alternative approaches	To assess program implementation, ideally as it happens	To describe program outcomes
Sample Questions	What are the educational needs? What resources are available (e.g., expertise)? What barriers are there?	What are the potential approaches within our context?	What happened? What went well? What was unexpected? What did we learn?	What were the (a) positive, (b) negative, and (c) unintended outcomes? How sustainable is the program? Can the program be adopted by other educators?
Data	Surveys Interviews Demographic information of participants Document review	Literature review Consult experts Information from exemplary programs	Observation Stakeholder interviews (learners, faculty)	Surveys Program report Assessment of achievement of program objectives

Two uses of ABR are described: (a) as a way to generate knowledge and (b) as a way to disseminate results.[31] In this section, we examine some examples of ABR in MH and review briefly some of the challenges and opportunities of using ABR in MH.

A number of studies using ABR are described in the MH literature. Joseph et al.[78] and Green et al.[79] describe their experience using mask-making and comics, respectively, to gain novel understandings into professional development, while Shapiro[80] describes how medical students made films to express their understandings of living with a chronic illness. One of the advantages of ABR is that it focuses on the subjective nature of experience and uses an interpretive philosophy of knowledge production. Participants are invited to get closer to their subjective experiences and their associated emotions. Through the creative process, learners' experiences are translated and made available to others.

My own experience of inviting learners to reflect on their clinical experiences of working in a multidisciplinary healthcare team by making a piece of art was very rewarding.[81] I initially offered the assignment to give learners with non-science backgrounds an opportunity to use their prior learning and was surprised when students with science backgrounds engaged just as enthusiastically. Students submitted a range of artwork, including music, poetry, collage, sculpture, and short film. Another example is given by Joseph et al.[78] In this study, the team used Gilligan's listening guide[82] and Kress and van Leeuwen's visual grammar[83] to help interpret students' masks. The listening guide uses a stepwise approach to help researchers hear and analyze multiple voices present in an individual's statements.[82] These voices can include perceptions of self, relationships with others, cultural voices, political views, and so on. The researcher listens for different elements of voice to hear what is being expressed or silenced within the sentences. Visual rhetoric examines the visual designs in artifacts to identify and analyze the culturally specific messages conveyed by the artist.[83] In my study, we used Gardener's entry points to look at the different ways in which we can enter into learning.[84] Other tools commonly used include SHOWeD methods used in photovoice to analyze photos (see, e.g., Patton[85] or Rose's critical visual methodology[86]). SHOWeD is a mnemonic: What did you See here? What is really Happening here? How does this relate to Our lives? Why does this problem, concern, or strength Exist? What can we Do about it?

One of the challenges using ABR is finding ways to appraise it. Boydell et al.,[31] in a review of ABR in health research, noted that researchers often drew on quality qualitative approaches such as independent coding, interrater agreement, regular team meetings, and debriefing to indicate trustworthiness of the work. Education researchers thinking of engaging with ABR can also provide in-depth descriptions of the study's context and intervention and the rationale underpinning their choice of intervention and analytic strategy. A specific challenge working with ABR is that ethical issues such as consent, privacy, and ownership tend to be compounded when extending learning beyond the traditional teacher–student dyad to include patients and others. Shapiro describes in detail some of the ethical dilemmas his team faced when making patient videos with students.[80]

A second role for ABR is that it offers an engaging means of presenting research findings. This may sound strange to those familiar with clinical conference presentations, but it is not un-common, at education and qualitative research conferences, for researchers to present a study in the form of a play or poem. For more local use, displaying or presenting students' artwork is a pow-erful vehicle to generate discussion with local faculty about the value of MH. Increasingly exhibitions such as White Coat, Warm Heart (Canadian Conference of Medical Education) and the Body Electric (International Conference on Residency Education) are common at medical education meetings. To date descriptions of using ABR as a medium of dissemination are rather limited in the medical education literature. Reports typically describe the presen-tation, exhibition, performance, or installation and gauge audience reaction and postperformance discussions.[87,88] Feedback from stakeholders often forms part of the process of documenting the project's significance, rigor, and originality.[89] Impact is embodied within the research itself rather than generated subsequently.

Displaying artwork plays an important role in extending health conversations beyond academia. By inviting our patients and communities to share in knowledge production and dissemination, ABR fulfills a critical role in MH as discursive, making scholarship more accessible to multiple audiences.

One of the particular advantages of ABR within MH is that its focus is to suggest new (and multiple) ways to view educational and health phenomena.[74] Too often our selection of methods is tied to knowledge-building tools that are available to us—we seek what we know how to find.[74] ABR as a form of expression is a powerful and underutilized means to evidence the value of MH education that provides a means to extend our understanding of evaluation and research beyond numbers and themed sound bites. Meaning-making, in a holistic sense, involves numbers and text but it also involves image, gesture, touch, and sound. Adopting ABR frees MH from science-imposed values and has the potential to enrich MH evaluation in ways that are more consistent with the scholarly and philosophical roots of the humanities. It is also in keeping with more complex modalities of evaluation and the constructivist paradigm of contemporary medical education research.

Conclusion

In this chapter, I highlighted some of the challenges and ways teachers and researchers of MH have addressed the topical issue of evaluation. Thirty-five years ago, a group of physicians, writers, and philosophers sat down to discuss the relationship between medicine and humanities as healing arts.[90] One of its members summarized the ensuing dialogue as a conversation between Apollo and Dionysis. Decades later, the conversation continues. Nothing about human experience and understanding or even the teaching and practice of medicine is straightforward. There is, however, a tendency to seek resolution, or the "right answer." Here I suggest that resolution or solutions are *not* what we seek. Rather, it is the very tensions between two opposing perspectives that is productive. Relating this to models of program evaluation, Bertalanffy[91] notes that equilibrium in a system can mean that nothing is changing—it could, in fact, represent a system that is dying. In contrast, an active system is one in which the elements are in balance—or perhaps even going in opposite directions, but active nonetheless. We can offer our residents an array of tools, options, and resources that help them construct new knowledge in rigorous yet creative ways. Increasingly, in the field of MH, this means combining evaluation and research methods which acknowledges their subjective and objective impressions, their hearts and minds. Importantly, we can encourage approaches to evaluation that honor the process of "drawing out value" from events (turning events into meaningful learning experiences) and that focus on the individual rather than attempting generalizations.

Acknowledgments

Many thanks to Profs. Alan Bleakley and Tim Dornan for their helpful feedback.

References

1. Doll WE Jr, Trueit D. Complexity and the health care professions. *J Eval Clin Pract.* 2010;16(4):841–848.
2. Nietzsche FW. *The Birth of Tragedy.* New York: Oxford University Press; 2000.
3. Evans M. Reflections on the humanities in medical education. *Med Educ.* 2002;36(6):508–513.
4. ACGME. *Glossary of terms.* Accreditation Council for Graduate Medical Education; 2013.
5. Ousager J, Johannessen H. Humanities in undergraduate medical education: a literature review. *Acad Med.* 2010;85(6):988–998.
6. Belling C. Commentary: sharper instruments: on defending the humanities in undergraduate medical education. *Acad Med.* 2010;85(6):938–940.

7. Charon R. Commentary: calculating the contributions of humanities to medical practice—motives, methods, and metrics. *Acad Med.* 2010;85(6):935–937.

8. Bleakley A. *Medical Humanities and Medical Education: How the Medical Humanities Can Shape Better Doctors.* Oxon: Routledge; 2015.

9. Shapiro J, Coulehan J, Wear D, Montello M. Medical humanities and their discontents: definitions, critiques, and implications. *Acad Med.* 2009;84(2):192–198.

10. Macnaughton J. The humanities in medical education: context, outcomes and structures. *Med Humanit.* 2000;26(1):23–30.

11. Shapiro J. Whither (whether) medical humanities? The future of humanities and arts in medical education. *J Learn Arts.* 2012;8(1).

12. Perry M, Maffulli N, Willson S, Morrissey D. The effectiveness of arts-based interventions in medical education: a literature review. *Med Educ.* 2011;45(2):141–148.

13. Evans HM. Affirming the existential within medicine: medical humanities, governance, and imaginative understanding. *J Med Humanit.* 2008;29(1):55–59.

14. Petersen A, Bleakley A, Brömer R, Marshall R. The medical humanities today: humane health care or tool of governance? *J Med Humanit.* 2008;29(1):1–4.

15. Rees G. The ethical imperative of medical humanities. *J Med Humanit.* 2010;31(4):267–277.

16. Wachtler C, Lundin S, Troein M. Humanities for medical students? A qualitative study of a medical humanities curriculum in a medical school program. *BMC Med Educ.* 2006;6(1):16.

17. Arntfield SL, Slesar K, Dickson J, Charon R. Narrative medicine as a means of training medical students toward residency competencies. *Patient Educ Couns.* 2013;91(3):280–286.

18. Belling C. Metaphysical conceit: toward a harder medical humanities *Atrium.* 2006;3:1–5.

19. Dennhardt S, Apramian T, Lingard L, Torabi N, Arntfield S. Rethinking research in the medical humanities: a scoping review and narrative synthesis of quantitative outcome studies. *Med Educ.* 2016;50(3):285–299.

20. Cook DA. Twelve tips for evaluating educational programs. *Med Teach.* 2010;32(4):296–301.

21. Daykin N, Joss T. *Arts for Health and Wellbeing: An Evaluation Framework.* London: Public Health England; 2016.

22. Balmer DF, Rama JA, Athina Martimianakis M, Stenfors-Hayes T. Using data from program evaluations for qualitative research. *J Grad Med Educ*. 2016;8(5):773–774.

23. Glassick CE. Boyer's expanded definitions of scholarship, the standards for assessing scholarship, and the elusiveness of the scholarship of teaching. *Acad Med*. 2000;75(9):877–880.

24. Beckman TJ, Cook DA. Developing scholarly projects in education: a primer for medical teachers. *Med Teach*. 2007;29(2–3): 210–218.

25. Malterud K. Qualitative research: standards, challenges, and guidelines. *Lancet*. 2001;358(9280):483–488.

26. Carter SM, Little M. Justifying knowledge, justifying method, taking action: epistemologies, methodologies, and methods in qualitative research. *Qual Health Res*. 2007;17(10):1316–1328.

27. Kuper A, Lingard L, Levinson W. Critically appraising qualitative research. *BMJ*. 2008;337:a1035.

28. Leppink J, Pérez-Fuster P. What is science without replication? *Perspect Med Educ*. 2016;5(6):320–322.

29. Higgins JP, Green S. *Cochrane Handbook for Systematic Reviews of Interventions*. Vol. 4. Hoboken, NJ: John Wiley; 2011.

30. Booth A. Searching for qualitative research for inclusion in systematic reviews: a structured methodological review. *Syst Rev*. 2016;5(1):1.

31. Wilczynski NL, Marks S, Haynes RB. Search strategies for identifying qualitative studies in CINAHL. *Qual Health Res*. 2007;17(5):705–710.

32. Walters LA, Wilczynski NL, Haynes RB. Developing optimal search strategies for retrieving clinically relevant qualitative studies in EMBASE. *Qual Health Res*. 2006;16(1):162–168.

33. Haidet P, Jarecke J, Adams NE, et al. A guiding framework to maximise the power of the arts in medical education: a systematic review and metasynthesis. *Med Educ*. 2016;50(3):320–331.

34. Kidd MG, Connor JT. Striving to do good things: teaching humanities in Canadian medical schools. *J Med Humanit*. 2008;29(1):45–54.

35. Boydell KM, Gladstone BM, Volpe T, Allemang B, Stasiulis E. The production and dissemination of knowledge: a scoping review of arts-based health research. *Qual Soc Res*. 2012;13.1.

36. Kuper A. Literature and medicine: a problem of assessment. *Acad Med*. 2006;81(10):S128–S137.

37. Cowen VS, Kaufman D, Schoenherr L. A review of creative and expressive writing as a pedagogical tool in medical education. *Med Educ.* 2016;50(3):311–319.

38. Schwartz AW, Abramson JS, Wojnowich I, Accordino R, Ronan EJ, Rifkin MR. Evaluating the impact of the humanities in medical education. *Mt Sinai J Med.* 2009;76(4):372–380.

39. Dornan T, Kelly M. What use is qualitative research? *Med Educ.* 2017;51(1):7–9.

40. Bearman M, Dawson P. Qualitative synthesis and systematic review in health professions education. *Med Educ.* 2013;47(3): 252–260.

41. Hannes K, Booth A, Harris J, Noyes J. Celebrating methodological challenges and changes: reflecting on the emergence and importance of the role of qualitative evidence in Cochrane reviews. *Syst Rev.* 2013;2(1):84.

42. Kelly M, Reid H, Bennett D, Yardley S, Dornan T. Introduction to qualitative evidence synthesis. Gold Foundation. http://www. gold-foundation.org/programs/research/mtl/introduction-qualitative-evidence-synthesis/. Accessed July 30, 2017.

43. Merriam SB. *Case Study Research in Education: A Qualitative Approach.* San Francisco: Jossey-Bass; 1988.

44. Baxter P, Jack S. Qualitative case study methodology: study design and implementation for novice researchers. *Qual Rep.* 2008;13(4):544–559.

45. Flyvbjerg B. Five misunderstandings about case-study research. *Qual Inq.* 2006;12(2):219–245.

46. Mennin S. Complexity and health professions education. *J Eval Clin Pract.* 2010;16(4):835–837.

47. Jorm C, Roberts C. Using complexity theory to guide medical school evaluations. *Acad Med.* 2017.

48. Frye AW, Hemmer PA. Program evaluation models and related theories: AMEE Guide No. 67. *Med Teach.* 2012;34(5): e288–e299.

49. Martin GP, McKee L, Dixon-Woods M. Beyond metrics? Utilizing "soft intelligence" for healthcare quality and safety. *Soc Sci Med.* 2015;142:19–26.

50. Jasani SK, Saks NS. Utilizing visual art to enhance the clinical observation skills of medical students. *Med Teach.* 2013;35(7):e1327–e1331.

51. Naghshineh S, Hafler JP, Miller AR, et al. Formal art observation training improves medical students' visual diagnostic skills. *J Gen Intern Med.* 2008;23(7):991–997.

52. Dolev JC, Friedlaender LK, Braverman IM. Use of fine art to enhance visual diagnostic skills. *JAMA.* 2001;286(9):1020–1021.

53. Kirklin D, Duncan J, McBride S, Hunt S, Griffin M. A cluster design controlled trial of arts-based observational skills training in primary care. *Med Educ.* 2007;41(4):395–401.

54. Rees C, Sheard C, Davies S. The development of a scale to measure medical students' attitudes towards communication skills learning: the Communication Skills Attitude Scale (CSAS). *Med Educ.* 2002;36(2):141–147.

55. Stanley Budner N. Intolerance of ambiguity as a personality variable. *J Pers.* 1962;30(1):29–50.

56. Geller G, Tambor ES, Chase GA, Holtzman NA. Measuring physicians' tolerance for ambiguity and its relationship to their reported practices regarding genetic testing. *Med Care.* 1993;31(11):989–1001.

57. Klugman CM, Peel J, Beckmann-Mendez D. Art rounds: teaching interprofessional students visual thinking strategies at one school. *Acad Med.* 2011;86(10):1266–1271.

58. Graham J, Benson LM, Swanson J, Potyk D, Daratha K, Roberts K. Medical humanities coursework is associated with greater measured empathy in medical students. *Am J Med.* 2016;129(12):1334–1337.

59. Artino AR Jr, La Rochelle JS, Dezee KJ, Gehlbach H. Developing questionnaires for educational research: AMEE Guide No. 87. *Med Teach.* 2014;36(6):463–474.

60. Glaser KM, Markham FW, Adler HM, McManus PR, Hojat M. Relationships between scores on the Jefferson Scale of Physician Empathy, patient perceptions of physician empathy, and humanistic approaches to patient care: a validity study. *Med Sci Monit.* 2007;13(7):CR291–CR294.

61. Hojat M, Mangione S, Kane GC, Gonnella JS. Relationships between scores of the Jefferson Scale of Physician Empathy (JSPE) and the Interpersonal Reactivity Index (IRI). *Med Teach.* 2005;27(7):625–628.

62. Krupat E, Rosenkranz SL, Yeager CM, Barnard K, Putnam SM, Inui TS. The practice orientations of physicians and patients: the

effect of doctor–patient congruence on satisfaction. *Patient Educ Couns.* 2000;39(1):49–59.

63. Haidet P, Dains JE, Paterniti DA, et al. Medical student attitudes toward the doctor–patient relationship. *Med Educ.* 2002;36(6):568–574.

64. Kirkpatrick D. Evaluation of training. In: Craig R, Bittel L, eds. *Training and Development Handbook.* New York: McGraw-Hill; 1967:87–112.

65. Wilkes M, Bligh J. Evaluating educational interventions. *BMJ.* 1999;318(7193):1269.

66. Yardley S, Dornan T. Kirkpatrick's levels and education "evidence." *Med Educ.* 2012;46(1):97–106.

67. Moreau KA. Has the new Kirkpatrick generation built a better hammer for our evaluation toolbox? *Med Teach.* 2017;39(9): 999–1001.

68. Cook DA, West CP. Perspective: reconsidering the focus on "outcomes research" in medical education: a cautionary note. *Acad Med.* 2013;88(2):162–167.

69. Kirkpatrick JD, Kirkpatrick WK. *Kirkpatrick's Four Levels of Training Evaluation.* Alexandria, VA: Association for Talent Development; 2016.

70. Pluye P, Hong QN. Combining the power of stories and the power of numbers: mixed methods research and mixed studies reviews. *Annu Rev Public Health.* 2013;35(1):29–45.

71. Glaser B, Strauss A. Grounded theory: the discovery of grounded theory. *Sociology.* 1967;12:27–49.

72. Charmaz K. *Constructing Grounded Theory: A Practical Guide Through Qualitative Analysis.* Thousand Oaks, CA: Pine Forge Press; 2006.

73. Atkinson P, Pugsley L. Making sense of ethnography and medical education. *Med Educ.* 2005;39(2):228–234.

74. Ng SL, Bisaillon L, Webster F. Blurring the boundaries: using institutional ethnography to inquire into health professions education and practice. *Med Educ.* 2017;51(1):51–60.

75. Dowling M. From Husserl to van Manen: a review of different phenomenological approaches. *Int J Nurs Stud.* 2007;44(1):131–142.

76. Finlay L. Debating phenomenological methods. *Hermen Phenomenol Educ.* 2012;4:17–37.

77. Dewey J. *Experience and Education.* New York: Simon & Schuster; 2007.

78. Bleakley A. Stories as data, data as stories: making sense of narrative inquiry in clinical education. *Med Educ*. 2005;39(5):534–540.
79. Charon R. At the membranes of care: stories in narrative medicine. *Acad Med*. 2012;87(3):342.
80. Clandinin DJ, Cave MT, Berendonk C. Narrative inquiry: a relational research methodology for medical education. *Med Educ*. 2017;51(1):89–96.
81. Atkins S, Roberts C, Hawthorne K, Greenhalgh T. Simulated consultations: a sociolinguistic perspective. *BMC Med Educ*. 2016;16. http://www.biomedcentral.com/1472-6920/16/16. Accessed July 30, 2017.
82. Gee JP. *An Introduction to Discourse Analysis: Theory and Method*. New York: Routledge; 2014.
83. Hodges BD, Martimianakis MA, McNaughton N, Whitehead C. Medical education . . . meet Michel Foucault. *Med Educ*. 2014;48(6):563–571.
84. Creswell JW, Poth CN. *Qualitative Inquiry and Research Design: Choosing Among Five Approaches*. London: SAGE; 2017.
85. Patton MQ. *Qualitative Research*. New York: Wiley Online Library; 2005.
86. Kumagai A. The Family Centered Experience: using patient narratives, student reflections, and discussions to teach about illness and care. *Behav Sci Med Educ*. 2005;11:73–77.
87. Kumagai AK. A conceptual framework for the use of illness narratives in medical education. *Acad Med*. 2008;83(7):653–658.
88. Kumagai AK. The patient's voice in medical education: The Family Centered Experience Program. *Virtual Mentor*. 2009;11(3):228.
89. Kumagai AK, Murphy EA, Ross PT. Diabetes stories: use of patient narratives of diabetes to teach patient-centered care. *Adv Health Sci Educ*. 2009;14(3):315.
90. Charmaz K. *Constructing Grounded Theory: A Practical Guide Through Qualitative Research*. London: SAGE; 2006.
91. Kumagai AK, Wear D. "Making strange": a role for the humanities in medical education. *Acad Med*. 2014;89(7):973–977.
92. Frechtling JA. *Logic Modeling Methods in Program Evaluation*. San Francisco: John Wiley; 2007.
93. Daykin N, Joss T. Arts for Health and Wellbeing: An Evaluation Framework. https://www.gov.uk/government/publications/

arts-for-health-and-wellbeing-an-evaluation-framework. Published 2016. Accessed July 30, 2017.

94. Stufflebeam DL. The CIPP model for evaluation. In: Kellaghan T, Stufflebeam D, eds. *The International Handbook of Educational Evaluation*. New York: Springer; 2003:31–62.

11

How to Fund and Promote Arts-Based Initiatives in Postgraduate Medical Education

ROBERT PIERRE TOMAS†

Reality Check

Even the best ideas die (or thrive) in implementation. To develop programs in medical humanities, is it enough to be a passionate, dedicated medical educator? Is it enough to believe that health humanities exposure and teaching are essential in medical education and, indeed, the medical profession? Is it enough to have heard Rita Charon present, to have subscribed to *Arts Medica*, to have attended Alan Bleakley's conferences in the UK, and to have a shelf-full of books (like this one) about the medical humanities? Well, no. There is one element that is absolutely necessary and the very one no one wants to talk about: money.

If you happen to be a confident new academic program lead in the university setting and have weekly brunches with your dean, then you may not have to worry about it. If, however, you are like most of your colleagues—an overworked, medical professional involved in the medical humanities for love not money—things may not be that easy. This chapter is not meant to be a complete "how to" fundraising tool but rather a collection of tips and suggestions; some of them may seem too basic for you, but some may reveal overlooked opportunities.

This will be a reality check.

The Problem with Change

"Change is unavoidable, growth is optional"—this "motivational" line is printed on T-shirts, coffee mugs, and mouse pads and resurfaces constantly in the form of Facebook memes. It would suggest that *Homo Sapiens* as a species embraces change. Except . . . this is not true. Of all the qualities that human beings value, the most cherished one is the exact opposite—the status quo. Change makers are outliers, rebels, outcasts. The majority of us value steady progress that does not threaten established structures. Change is threatening, and threats lead to resistance. Educational institutions are no different, and rocking the boat is not always encouraged. You will encounter resistance, but do not be discouraged. Eventually change sticks and ultimately is even welcomed.

So what can be done?

First, it is best to know what lies ahead: This is going to be challenging. The more conventional the prevailing intellectual mode of your institution, the harder it will be. There are no quick, quantitative studies proving your point. Instead, the strength of humanities lies in the qualitative realm. In order to become an effective change maker, you will have to have allies. Yes, some of them will be of the "slow and steady" persuasion. Enlist them for your cause, as they have discovered how to survive and thrive in the academic environment. Sometimes there will be setbacks, but setbacks are not the end of the road. So make sure to celebrate the small successes until they grow large. Most of all, keep going and do not lose your passion for the medical humanities.

To further illustrate the problem of change, let me introduce the concept of "learning anxiety."

It is best explained in an interview in the *Harvard Business Review*[1] with Edgar H. Schein, Sloan Fellows Professor of Management Emeritus at MIT's Sloan School of Management. Schein is a psychologist, and some of his early research involved US veterans who were prisoners of war (POWs) during the Korean conflict. The Korean prisoners' camps were brutal places, where brainwashing and indoctrination were standard fare. Surprisingly, despite the

POWs' traumatic experience, Schein shows that the anxiety levels of the POWs are similar to those experienced by any learners—be it people in the workplace (where they must adapt to a new culture/way of thinking/ new concepts), academics in the institution, where a new administration is drastically changing the ways of "doing business," or where whole new concepts/departments are introduced. Moreover, approximately 80% of these soldiers survived well by remaining passive. So resisting change is often protective, and you have to convince the passive and anxious protectors that new is not dangerous. This paints the landscape for the change maker: 80% of people whose minds you are trying to change will be passive; the remaining 20% will be highly anxious about the changes you are proposing. You will have to get it right *with their help.*

The Basics

There are two necessary elements before you get started: resources and a plan. By resources, I mean available materials including manpower (try to recruit possible supporters early on) and funds. The plan is the vision you have for your humanities program and a strategy for getting to that vision.

Evidence

In order to convince your institution's sceptics of the value of humanities, you will need evidence. This includes published studies, medical journal articles, descriptions of programs created at competing schools or medical institutions, the results of your own work, patient interviews, and feedback from other medical professionals—essentially anything that you can lay your hands on. (Every chapter of this book summarizes the evidence for including humanities teaching within postgraduate medical education. Use these references to promote the arts-based modality you wish to develop.) Having the evidence is the first part; disseminating it is the other. Strategically, share your evidence with your colleagues. Your "slow and steady" colleagues can be very useful here—essentially, sharing *your* ideas with others does not affect the way they operate. Have them forward the critical pieces (essential articles, published studies) to their networks and the powers that be. Start creating a "grassroots" awareness of the medical humanities as was suggested in chapter 1. Some small-scale examples of pilot programs in your department, within the resident doctors' community as well as among patients, are listed in Box 11.1.

You can use any other pilot program described in this book; just make sure you can deliver within your means (materials, people, and money).

BOX 11.1 Just Starting Up

Curate a film night in your hospital, for residents and patients, on medical topics. There is a plethora of suitable films listed elsewhere in this book. All you need to provide is a large enough room, a computer projector, and some "free" (more on that later Box 11.2) pizza. Make sure that all your pilot projects, their outcomes, feedback, and evaluations are collected on your website, Facebook group page, and your Twitter feed. To that end, implement very rigid brand guidelines. Refer to your planned program in a consistent way, so the name starts acquiring "brand equity" (a fancy way of saying that people will recognize it). For example, "Asklepios Medical Humanities Group presents its Monthly Film Night"; "At the latest screening of *Wit* presented by the Asklepios Medical Humanities Group . . ."; "Patients were enthusiastic about the latest initiative of the Asklepios Medical Humanities Group . . .," etc.).

Building awareness of your program increases your visibility, but it also makes it easier to fundraise for the further development of the program. The problem, again, is money—and building awareness requires it.

Funding

At first, your own *voluntary* (i.e., unpaid) commitment is a given. Trust me: from the perspective of over 20 years in non-profit fundraising, the last thing donors want to fund is salaries. The help of your volunteer fellow travellers is crucial. For example, remember that website you need to create? Maybe some of your colleagues or residents are web-savvy enough to build it for you.

There is no better donation than acquiring the things you need for *free*. Meeting space, curatorial efforts, and office supplies—all can be acquired through exchange, bartering, and the voluntary contributions of your friends and allies.

Exchange services far and wide; for example, provide art school students with access to anatomy classes for their drawing sessions. In exchange, enlist their help to create a seminar on the arts for students, patients, or faculty and invite them to visual literacy sessions dedicated to the "close reading" of works of art. Bring a large group of your colleagues to a lecture on history of the plague at your local museum. Then invite that lecturer to do a presentation at your med school for patients and colleagues. Simply view your medical humanities efforts as resonating in the society at large and thus obtain the involvement from the local community to help prove to your powers that be that this work is needed.

Remember, you are implementing these grassroots strategies so the program (e.g., Asklepios Medical Humanities Group) gets off the ground see Box 11.2 for some examples, well before you ask your postgraduate dean and your chair for funding.

The crucial part of any fundraising is friend-raising. Fundraising is 100% based on forging relationships. As a doctor, you are called upon to form countless, therapeutic relationships with your patients. Granted, they involve strict boundaries (and, to this end,

BOX 11.2 With a Little Help from Your Friends

And then there is the "free" pizza! Simple solution? Have your friends over for dinner. Tell them that in lieu of flowers/gifts/bottles of wine, they should bring checks in an amount of their choosing, issued to the Asklepios Medical Humanities Group, c/o you. Congratulations: you have just raised the first $1,000 for your program. (It helps if not all of your friends are medical doctors. Maybe it's the feeling of "I've given at the office," but doctors on both sides of the Atlantic are rarely listed among the most generous of donors.)

There are different variants of this fundraising approach you could try—a fundraising BBQ on the campus of your medical school, coinciding conveniently with a lunch break; a "give your change to make change" collection at the hospital cafeteria or library (make sure to obtain appropriate approvals); a bake sale. Some of you are accomplished athletes: climbers, cyclists, runners. Approach your entire sports network to sponsor your climb/ride/run.

Try something different: at your film night (presented by the Asklepios Medical Humanities Group), auction off a piece of movie memorabilia stuck in your attic.

Come up with your own dramatic idea—after all, someone came up with the Ice Bucket Challenge for ALS.

never raise money directly from your patients!). However, they are based on mutual trust—just as fundraising relationships should be. So, when approaching donors, treat them as if they were your patients: respect them, say what you mean to say, and, in keeping with the very core values of medical humanities, *listen to them*! They may have even better ideas for you.

Incidentally, there is nothing wrong ethically if a former patient (given enough time has passed) were to approach you or your department and say: "I've heard wonderful things about the Asklepios Medical Humanities Group . . ." or "it helped me tremendously at the time and I would like to contribute to your program." You can even have pamphlets on the group's activities in your office or medical school offices. If not comfortable accepting donations, you can direct patients to your hospital or med school foundation (see later discussion). Remember to instruct them that they should be very specific as to where their donation is allocated—the foundation is obligated to honor the donor's wishes.

Why Me?

Many doctors bristle at the thought of having to do their own fundraising. The hospital and the university have their own foundation/advancement department with people *paid* and *trained* to do this. Keep in mind that hospital foundations' goals are established by the board of directors and hospital administration, usually under the catch-all umbrella of patient outcomes. To them it usually means raising funds for that new high-tech machine crucial to the "patient outcomes." Universities are all about "student experience," which usually means a new building. Remember: you are the agent of change challenging the status quo and will not initially be a priority for fundraisers. Try having lunch with your foundation head (or his or her deputy) and explain how the work of the Asklepios Humanities Group has had a demonstrable impact on "patient outcomes," including patient satisfaction. Keep track of anything written/published in the local press and mentions in the hospital and university newsletters about the work you are doing.

Ask them to schedule a meeting where you can present a PowerPoint on your goals, initiatives, and outcomes. Having them on your side does not guarantee that the foundation will raise money for your program, but at least you will get its benign neglect: non-interference in your small fundraising initiatives, *and*, if you are lucky, it will promote your efforts through a mention or a feature in the foundation's newsletter, circulated to all donors. Foundation members will also keep your program in mind should the ideal arts-motivated donor come along.

Resources (of the Human Kind)

As stated, because your volunteer services are a given and salaries are the most difficult component of your program to raise money for, there is no question that you will have to eventually figure out how to pay for the remuneration of staff, especially administrative staff, when your program is well established. The first step is to create a budget. This very word strikes fear in the hearts of competent medical women and men. It is, however, not that difficult (see Box 11.3).

Look at all the efforts of Asklepios Medical Humanities Group and list the approximate value.

If you hold more events, your annual or semester budget will be a multiple of those charges and may include a speakers' fees,

---

BOX 11.3 Sample Budget: A Film Night for Patients

Room rental for a movie night for patients $200
AV equipment (offered for free by Jack Smith)
    would cost to rent $350
5 boxes of pizza, 2 vegetarian, 3 omnivorous $70
2 Volunteer ushers ($10/hr for 3 hrs) $60
Copying of satisfaction evaluation materials $10
Posters and e-mail publicity in the hospital $35
Volunteered administrative time (7 hrs at $10/hr) $70

their transportation/parking and per diem, as well as any other expenses. Of course, your real budget will not list the toppings on the pizza—it is merely an illustration that shows you have to anticipate—and budget for—many contingencies.

Even when most of what you achieve is performed by volunteers, do not forget to include staff costs in your program budget, because you have no guarantee that you will always have volunteers—including yourself.

Remember not to overburden and burn out your volunteers, including yourself. When holding an event seems insurmountable with present resources, maybe it is time to pause and re-evaluate.

When raising money for your program, budget in hand, do not overlook opportunities such as summer jobs for students/electives for residents co-funded by federal/national and state governments, targeted arts grants from municipalities and other levels of government, potential stipends available from your professional associations, educational development funds at your medical school, and other such sources. Finally, many private foundations will provide "seed money" to get a program started, including some salary provisions. Maybe you can negotiate a secondment agreement with another department/faculty. This model is successfully deployed by multiple United Way/Community Chest campaigns, where an employee is seconded (detached) from his or her original position and he or she performs duties related to the campaign/program, while the salary is still being paid by the original employer.

For example, at the University of Toronto, the Medical Illustrator in Residence was permitted by her health sciences medical illustration faculty to teach seminars and supervise residents for graphic medicine electives. Although this position was unfunded, it gave her opportunities to build up professional networks, and the work led to publications that were extremely helpful in creating her promotion dossier. Emphasizing the mutual benefits of this work to other academics can be very fruitful. Her story (quoted by permission) is given in Box 11.4.

BOX 11.4 Second(ed) Hand Help

I have a full-time faculty position in Biomedical Communications (BMC) at the University of Toronto. Our degree is offered through the Institute of Medical Science. Many of our faculty and students are involved in research/collaborations with clinicians and researchers from the faculty of medicine, and BMC has deep historical ties to the faculty.

When I presented the illustrator in residence opportunity to my program director, we agreed that the role would

- Constitute valuable professional development for me and complement the research and teaching I already do within BMC (in graphic medicine and visual communication for medical and patient education);
- Provide ideas, connections, and experiences that could contribute directly to my growth as a researcher and educator within BMC;
- Provide yet another connection for our program to the faculty of medicine, a relationship we are eager to nurture.

The illustrator-in-residence role included spending some time each week involved in, among other things, giving seminars and supervising students. This was an informal agreement. This was not a huge departure for BMC, as it's the nature of our profession that we engage in collaborative, interdisciplinary projects, and most of our faculty collaborate with researchers and clinicians throughout the university.

So, in a sense, my home program "donates" some of my time. In return, it obtains professional development for one of its faculty members, which translates into indirect benefits for BMC itself.

The "Magic" of Major Gifts

There are many definitions of what a major gift is, but, in all instances, the actual amount is fully contingent on the size of your program and its needs. For the purpose of this book, a major gift is any gift that will have a *transformational* impact on your program. If you are just starting, receiving $1,000 from one donor will be transformational: it will pay for all those pizzas and new business cards for you. A $5,000 gift to a fledgling program will allow for creation of a professionally designed website (with a DONATE HERE button at the top of the page—something many organizations forget about). Once the program is up and running, the transformation will come from a $1.5 million endowed chair. No matter the amount, major gifts are the holy grail of fundraising, because they presumably provide the biggest "bang-for-buck" ratio. Rather than getting $10 each from 100 people, you are getting the whole $1,000 from one person/ a private foundation/corporation. Strictly speaking, a corporate gift would be seen as a sponsorship (a business deal) rather than a charitable gift, but since Asklepios Medical Humanities Group has no tax-exempt status (yet!) and cannot issue tax receipts, the distinction is moot. So one gift versus 100 means 99 fewer thank-you notes to write and 99 fewer reports to the donor about what you did with the money. Nonetheless, you must be very careful negotiating major gifts. Ten-dollar gifts rarely come with strings attached; $1,000 gifts usually do.

In the case of individual major gifts, people often have the idea that they know better how it should be spent. Say a donor has a son who is an aspiring filmmaker and has just finished his most recent feature on a vaguely medical theme. The donor thinks the Film Night presented by the Asklepios Medical Humanities Group is the perfect forum to premiere the masterpiece. If you accept the money with this proviso, you may have to present the less than artful movie, potentially jeopardizing the reputation of your program.

Be clear on what you can and cannot offer (even with some extra funding). "Mission drift" occurs when you embark on activities not warranted by your mandate and not planned by you but required as a condition of a major gift agreement. If the threat of mission drift is real and imminent, you are best to refuse the gift, as much as that may hurt.

For the reasons outlined here, it is best practice to have a written agreement with the individual major gift donor. Foundations and corporations will insist on one.

A major gift agreement is not strictly a legal agreement—the gift has to be voluntary and can be revoked, so it is not legally binding. It is, however, honor-binding. If you have agreed to fulfill a certain donor's requirements, you should do so in a timely and transparent manner. Remember: donors have the money you need. You and the Asklepios Medical Humanities Group only have your reputations—and your honor.

The "safest" major gifts in terms of avoiding mission drift are grants that come from private (and quasi-governmental) foundations. (A list of funders in the United States, Canada, and the United Kingdom is provided in the appendix.) In essence, they lay it all out on the table during the application process. They inform you what conditions your program must meet, what documents need to be submitted, what constitutes acceptable expenditures from the grant for operations, and what the reporting requirements are. If you ever applied for a research grant, you will be familiar with this process. If you have not, do read the instructions carefully and, to avoid disappointment, talk on the phone or in person with a foundation officer to clarify some grey areas. There is nothing worse than putting a lot of work into an application deemed ineligible.

There is another reason to talk to the agency's grant officer. Remember the friend-raising aspect of fundraising? Many applications severely limit the number of pages/words/characters in their templates. This can be circumvented by painting a much broader picture with many more examples during a meeting with the granting agency personnel or even a "site visit"—an invitation to attend a screening, presented by the Asklepios Medical Humanities Group.

In the case of major gifts received from corporations, very few of them will come as a charitable contribution. In the industrialized world, corporate charitable giving *is manifold less* than the funds spent by those corporations to promote their corporate social responsibility (i.e., charitable giving).[2] In other words, those glossy, colourful corporate social responsibility reports cost more to print than the actual gifts given. As a result, most of your funds will be in sponsorship agreements. They will not be charitable donations; they will be business arrangements, where you will have to deliver as well. You will get the money, and the corporation will receive acknowledgement, recognition, participation opportunities, or anything else you can negotiate. Be prepared to offer a write-up on your website or Twitter-feed, logo placement on your materials, and, increasingly important for corporations, volunteering opportunities for their employees. Of course when dealing with the pharmaceutical industry, do refer to established guidelines specified by your postgraduate medical education office.

The Art of Saying Thank You

One of the most popular mistaken beliefs about fundraising is that it is "just like sales." True, there is an element of cultivating (advertising), soliciting (making a sale), and receiving money (getting payment), but here the similarities end. Payment is the end of the sales transaction (after all, warranty service is the portfolio of another department). In fundraising, the payment is merely one of many steps in the developing relationship. That is why stewardship (or the art of saying "thank you") is so important. First, do not ever worry about over-thanking your donors. Eventually, their modesty will kick in, and, if you are really overdoing it, they will tell you to stop. Much more dangerous is not thanking them enough. In many cases, you may have an electronic system (say, a "Donate Now" button on your website) equipped with an ability to immediately send a generic thank you letter/tax receipt. *This is a start but it is never enough.* Try to find time to call donors and thank them personally or ask one of the trainees to do so, to show how their gift has impacted their career. Remember: a positive association with the first donation is likely to result in a follow-up gift. It bears repeating that fundraising is all about relationships. You need to develop them. So, with the assistance of your colleagues, students, and residents, inform your donors of your progress. Tell them exactly how their money was spent (and "we've put it in the general fund and lost track of it" is not the right way to do it). Give them sample resident evaluations with a summary of comments. Try to figure out the granular cost of your program elements (e.g., free pizza for the film night, printing of brochures, cost of one participant attending a workshop, cost of the supervision of one resident, etc.). Have these numbers on the ready and use them in proportion of your donor's contribution (e.g., "Your generous gift of $2,000 allowed me to personally supervise four residents in deepening their knowledge of medical humanities"). Donors want to know what their real-life impact is and what changes occurred because of their donation.

Similarly, donor recognition should not be limited to plaques crowding hospital and university walls. These are fine, but in many cases, donors do not really want them (be sure to ask about their preferences). Instead, *experiential* recognition is much more effective. Invite important donors to help you curate an art show or movie night, or invite them to a meet and greet with a visiting fellow, prominent author, or lecturer they admire. Ask them to sit on the jury of a student/resident arts contest. This type of recognition will deepen your relationship much more than any plaque would.

A Special Case: Artist in Residence Programs

One of the fastest ways to give some prominence to the Asklepios Medical Humanities Group is to set up an artist in residence (AIR) program (see Box 11.5). It works on several levels. If chosen properly, the artist can bring name recognition to the program and to your group. Artists in residence also resonate and interact with a much broader audience than most of your other programs. It is highly unlikely that your hospital administrator would visit your weekend workshop on reflective writing; however, he or she may be more likely to come see what the commotion is when your poet in residence sets up an instant poetry booth in the lobby. The range of possibilities is quite large, and most artists are willing to take on a prospect of steady albeit modest pay in exchange for sharing their artistic insights and doing some workshops. It could be a photographer in residence, taking pictures (with consent) of patients as they are leaving the hospital after a successful treatment (keep these activities upbeat). Of course, this is a new area in hospitals and many medical schools, so expect some resistance (including "risk analysis"). Most importantly, do not forget to gather feedback, such as post-workshop evaluations or a blog, accessible to patients/ participants on your website. Never forget about the task of gathering evidence for your program. Your artist in residence will have to prepare an annual report for funders, but recruit him or her to produce creative summaries for broader distribution.

The next part of our conversation may be considered by some to be a delicate topic. Hospitals are places of healing. By their very nature, they are also places of death. However, this, too, can create possibilities for your program. Funding, or even endowing an AIR program to commemorate a loved one who was an artist or admired art, can be one of the most meaningful ways to keep the thought of them alive.

If you encounter a donor interested in such commemoration, an AIR program can be ideal: it has broad appeal, it is meaningful and creative, and it has the halo effect of a sophisticated remembrance—something the donor will enjoy much more than a dusty plaque in one of the side corridors.

AIR programs also offer a great publicity opportunity—so do not hesitate to invite your local paper, radio station, or TV station to a painting workshop held by your artist for patients on the ward.

BOX 11.5 The Best Gifts Don't Cost a Thing

Would the gallery representing a famous painter be willing to participate? Would a publisher consider supporting a poet's contribution to the program? Would a literary magazine be interested in showcasing the work of your writer in residence? Could you maybe interest your local museum/music school/department of literature/MFA program in sharing the administration of this program (which not only lessens the expense but also broadens the reach)?

Make it obvious to the hospital or university that this type of publicity is very good, thus strengthening your hand in further program development.

Make your reach as broad as possible.

Again, keep your medical school's/hospital's foundation abreast of any queries and developments as you go along—you never know what might catch someone's eye.

The important part to remember is that AIR programs are not meant to replace or displace other activities but rather to enhance them and to highlight innovations in your hospital or medical school.

Keep Your Eyes on the Prize

Much of what this chapter has discussed will seem like drudgery or overwhelming or both. I know it first hand; there are easier ways of making a living than fundraising. What you must protect in this process is your passion for the cause. Know why you are doing it. Your objective should be to develop the humanities program to the point where your medical school/postgraduate office/hospital can no longer ignore it. In an ideal world, you would have an academic merit fund, protecting the time you decide to dedicate to the

Asklepios Medical Humanities Group. Depending on the relationship with your medical school dean/departmental chair and your own prominence within that academic environment, it may never be too early to request hard funding for your time. Write to humanities leads and directors at other schools and residency programs and ask them to share strategies—even the proposals they submitted. Networking resources are supplied in chapter 1. If you feel (or know for a fact) that your name alone does not yet carry enough clout, strike alliances with more prominent/senior colleagues and share your passion for the project with them. Try and remove your ego from the process—it's only natural that your new allies will want a part of the "glory pie." Remember the Roman saying: "Success has many fathers; failure is an orphan." It is well documented elsewhere in this book that medical humanities teaching within residency will improve patient outcomes, physician well-being, and communication between healthcare professionals and their patients and families. It may certainly protect many professionals from work-related burnout and will definitely be a valuable learning experience for you, but, in the end, it will accomplish something even greater: it will be a transformative change in your educational institution. Always keep that in mind when you weary of asking for money and scheduling yet another working lunch. This may well be your legacy.

List of Lists

The following is a simple listing of things to remember when working on developing a medical humanities program and/or teaching within residency programs.

Never

- Miss an opportunity to thank a donor
- Forget that sometimes the simplest solutions are within your reach—if you do not have money to put on a workshop,

consider charging the participants a small fee; as you collect your daily latte from Starbucks/Costa/Tim Hortons, don't forget to ask the manager if he or she would be willing to donate coffee and snacks for your next film night; as you are paying fees to the faculty association/college of physicians and surgeons/specialty association, investigate any availability of grants for educational innovation/supports in-kind (use of space, use of equipment, distribution of leaflets/email/ listservs posts).

- Forget that pharma/industry support for seminars, conferences, and teaching opportunities must be discussed with your postgraduate medicine dean, as rules for "unrestricted grants" differ from school to school and internationally.
- Push your volunteers (and yourself) until you drop from fatigue, but also know the value of strategic retreat.
- Do anything in your fundraising activities that would not pass the "smell test" in your professional and daily life.
- Forget to rely on your sense of integrity. Don't burn bridges, if possible. Stick to your values and principles.
- Assume that your colleagues are against you (some of them might be, but that's another story). They may be anxious about the changes you are proposing, fear more work on their part, or be relying on passivity to "ride out" the new approach.

Always

- Ask for help when you need it. You will be surprised by who will actually say yes.
- Celebrate success. Any success. You will hear "no" more often than "yes," so you owe yourself and your partners those celebrations. Ask your residents to use social media and your website to share the news.
- Be consistent in your approach—do not offer "side deals" to some donors but not others—it always comes out, to everyone's embarrassment.

- Build the brand equity of your program—and guard it from imitators, no matter how flattering that might be ("based on the model developed by Asklepios Medical Humanities Group" should be an introduction to any "me-too" events).
- Keep your students, colleagues, and bosses appraised of your activities—you are not "beating your own drum"; you are creating a transformative program. Don't forget to keep donors in the loop too. Email them regularly with updates and ask them to join your event list-serves.
- Remember that fundraising is really about relationship building. The more you do it, the better you will get at it.
- Keep your eyes on the prize—helping to train humanistic, patient-centered physicians.
- Plan for succession. Your work with residents will produce the next cohort of educators willing to champion the medical humanities in clinical and learning settings.

References

1. Coutu, Diane L. "The Learning Anxiety." HBR Interview. *Harvard Business Review*, March 2002.
2. For some sobering examples, watch the documentary "Philanthropy, Inc." ©2009 http://castlewoodproductions.com/production/philanthropy-inc/, also available on YouTube.

Afterword

CRAIG IRVINE

On a Tuesday morning in mid-August 2016 at 7:55 AM I enter the inpatient service unit of the Family Medicine Residency Program at the New York Presbyterian Hospital to lead narrative medicine rounds, as I have every week for the past 15 years. I enter the conference room and find Jen and Silas (the two interns), Susana (a senior resident), and Maria (a senior medical student) seated at the long conference table, bent over their laptops, intently studying charts, placing orders—conducting the urgent business that will save patients' lives, attempt to ease their suffering, record their births and deaths. The other senior resident is with a patient who took a turn for the worse overnight. A few minutes later Edgar, the attending physician, enters, and I hand around the morning's reading, section 2 from "Elegy for My Father" by Mark Strand:[1]

Why did you travel?
Because the house was cold.
Why did you travel?
Because it is what I have always done between sunset and sunrise.
What did you wear?
I wore a blue suit, a white shirt, yellow tie, and yellow socks.
What did you wear?
I wore nothing. A scarf of pain kept me warm.
Who did you sleep with?
I slept with a different woman each night.
Who did you sleep with?

I slept alone. I have always slept alone.
Why did you lie to me?
I always thought I told the truth.
Why did you lie to me?
Because the truth lies like nothing else and I love the truth.
Why are you going?
Because nothing means much to me anymore.
Why are you going?
I don't know. I have never known.
How long shall I wait for you?
Do not wait for me. I am tired and I want to lie down.
Are you tired and do you want to lie down?
Yes, I am tired and I want to lie down.

Jen volunteers to read the poem aloud. When she finishes, I ask for two more volunteers, one to take the part of the questioner and the other to read the answers. I then ask the team to comment on what they have noticed in the poem.

Jen begins by discussing the differences between the first and second answers to each of the repeated questions. She notes that the second answers all seem to go deeper, to get closer to the truth. She relates this to her interviews with patients, saying that patients who are avoidant or who want to put the best face on things will often respond superficially to an initial query but will "open up" when a question is repeated.

Susana is not sure she agrees that the second answers are "more true." Both answers are true, she avers, but they describe different aspects of experience. Just because something is true on one level at one time but not on another level at another time does not make it false or superficial. One of the challenges for a clinician, Susana contends, is accepting the truth of seemingly contradictory answers.

Maria points to the poet's equivocal use of the word "lie." She puzzles over the relationships among the three meanings of the word. She notes that the poet's first use of "lie," in line 13, means "to speak falsely." This first "lie," however, immediately follows the two instances of the question, "Who did you sleep with?" The resonance of that question sounds in this first use of "lie," because "to lie with" is a synonym for "to sleep with" in both its literal (sleep) and figurative (sex) senses. The meaning of "lie" in the last three sentences, Maria continues, is "to put oneself into a horizontal position," but the ambiguity of the earlier uses of the word carries over, complicating its use here at the end of the poem.

Silas finds the greatest ambiguity in the sentence, "Because the truth lies like nothing else and I love the truth." "Does anyone have *any* idea what that means?" he asks. Edgar answers that he can't be sure but that he often finds that, when someone lies, it's for a reason. It's important to look for that reason—to look for what the lie reveals. Interrogating a "lie" can often reveal a deeper truth, he contends, than a simple, "straightforward" answer. Edgar adds that he likes the way the final question breaks the pattern, repeating what the respondent has just said in the form of a question, rather than just repeating the same question again. "I hear you," the interrogator seems to be saying, bringing their conversation to a close but in a way that still "contains" the ambiguity.

The team discusses the poem for 20 minutes, then I give them the following prompt: "Write about a time you had two answers to the same question." As usual, I encourage them to write out their responses spontaneously, without editing. At the four-minute mark I give them a one-minute warning, and when five minutes are up, I tell them to finish their last sentences. I remind them that anything that's shared in the room should remain confidential because they may be writing about patients, colleagues, or personal matters and encourage them not to preface before reading.

Silas reads first. He writes about having recently ended his relationship with a woman he'd lived with for several years. He's sure it was the right decision, and he's sure it wasn't. Susanna points to the way the intern's equivocal use of several terms expresses an ambiguity that mirrors the poet's use of "lie." Edgar points to the ways the intern's narrative represents the process of coming to terms with a decision—the way it moves back and forth, ebbs and flows, between competing, ever deepening interests. In this way the intern's piece, the attending contends, might be a profound representation of loss and regret and of the realization that there is often no "perfect" choice, always a price to be paid for every decision.

Susanna reads her response next. It's about a patient encounter in the primary care clinic the previous week, but Susanna writes in the present tense. The patient is a 40-year-old man with sickle cell disease, seeking an increase in his opioid pain medication. The patient reports that he has recently experienced an exacerbation of his symptoms; he has a history of drug abuse, and the resident is both sympathetic and skeptical. Maria points to the way Susanna powerfully represents her ambivalence by posing the question "Should I increase his pain medication?" not just twice but six times, moving back and forth between "Yes" and "No," much like Silas's piece did, though the subjects of the two pieces are completely different. Silas agrees, noting that he now recognizes that in both of their pieces each subsequent answer adds a level of complexity to each side of the decision without providing an easy resolution. Silas points out that the senior's use of present tense keenly expresses how this experience is still very much "with" her.

Maria reads, and I read, and Jen passes. Edgar reads last. His piece is about his mother, who is in a nursing home, suffering from Alzheimer's disease. Edgar's narrative is written as the transcript of a conversation, in which he asks his mother the same question again and again, receiving different answers each time. Some of the answers are clearly cogent, some clearly not, and some ambiguous. Halfway through his reading, Edgar begins to cry and finds it difficult to continue. He would like the rest to be heard, however, so he passes it to Susanna to finish reading. When Susanna finishes, I ask the team to take a moment before responding. We sit in silence for a minute, and then I ask Edgar if he would like to hear our reflections about his piece, or if he'd rather that we move on. He says he'd love to hear our thoughts. Jen remarks that she is struck by the rhythms of the conversation Edgar has represented—how they could be the rhythms of everyday speech between two people without cognitive deficits. Edgar's relationship with his mother,

Jen asserts, is expressed in those rhythms, more than in the details of what is said. This reminds Susanna that much of what is communicated by patients is conveyed nonverbally, or in the *forms* the verbal expressions take, not just the content. "Like a poem," she adds, looking at me and smiling.

The rhythms of everyday speech: how often we've heard laments about the ways these cadences are interrupted during clinical encounters. It's often said that the ability, or at least the desire, to relate *humanly* with patients is trained out of physicians by the time they graduate from residency. In a sense, all of the efforts described in this book are attempts to bring physicians into explicit, robust connection with their own and their patients' humanity. This is particularly important during residency training. Interns are arguably the most anxious physicians on the planet; the shift from medical school to residency is dramatic, as the young doctors suddenly feel the weight of responsibility for patients' lives. Residency is a time when most physicians turn away from anything that might "distract" them from acquiring the clinical scientific knowledge that they believe is the only thing that stands between them and catastrophic failure. Yet it is precisely for this reason that it is during residency, more than at any other point in medical training, that the health humanities should be incorporated into curricula. As the authors of this volume have argued, sound clinical practice requires more than the acquisition of clinical scientific knowledge. Much more.

It requires an understanding of "illness as a multifactorial process" and "attention to the social aspects of medicine" that social science education supports. It requires the ability "to face head-on the limits of medical knowledge" and "to engage with complex stories, ethical dilemmas and ambiguity" that theater and film foster. It requires a willingness to question and transform "perceptions of issues such as human rights, equity, illness, treatment, and the process of healing," enhanced through engagement with the visual arts. In order to care for others, one must not only master the pathophysiology of illness, disease, and disability but also understand their *meaning* both for the patient and for the provider—understanding that requires narrative competence. And if one's care is to reflect "appropriate core values," one must be able "to recognize and identify the ethical aspects of care and make difficult ethical decisions."

When our hour is up I say goodbye to the team and head for the door. As I leave the room, I can hear Jen begin to present the patient she admitted late yesterday: ". . .67-year-old female with HTN, smoking, DM, PAD but no known CAD. . . ." I know the form well, and I don't have to focus on the content, so what I hear most vividly is the fear in Jen's voice. I don't have to understand the numerous abbreviations to know that her patient is very ill. This is Jen's first month on the wards. She is young—so very young—and clearly overwhelmed. She is, however, in good hands. This team knows a great deal about facing fear together. They know that becoming a doctor is not about hiding from their feelings, their vulnerabilities, their all-too-human bodies. The doctor and philosopher Emmanuel Levinas writes, "The doctor is an a priori principle of human morality."[2] To become a doctor—a lifelong work—is to become ever more human. Only the humanities can teach us what this means.

References

1. Strand, Mark. New Selected Poems. New York: Alfred A. Knopf, 2007.
2. Levinas, Emmanuel. Totality and Infinity: An Essay on Exteriority. Translated by Alphonso Lingis. Pittsburgh, PA: Duquesne University Press; 1969.

Appendix

Suggested Readings and Resources

Chapter 1: Why Are the Heath Humanities Relevant (and Vital) in Postgraduate Medical Education?

Suggested Reading

Jones, Therese, Wear, Delese, and Friedman, Lester D., eds. *Health Humanities Reader*. New Brunswick, NJ: Rutgers University Press; 2014.

Peterkin, Allan, and Brett-MacLean, Pamela. eds. *Keeping Reflection Fresh: A Practical Guide for Clinical Educators*. Kent: Kent State University Press; 2016.

Health/Medical Humanities Associations with Annual Conferences and Workshops

Association for Medical Humanities (UK): https://amh.ac.uk/
American Society of Bioethics and Humanities (US): www.asbh.org
Canadian Association of Health Humanities (Canada): www.cahh.ca

Web Resources

http://medhum.med.nyu.edu/
A rich list of readings/resources/curricula.

List-Serves

Use these emails to join these two very helpful lists. Educators often share teaching strategies/curricula upon request.
healthhum@simplelists.com (US list)
ahssm-came@mailman.srv.ualberta.ca (Canadian list)

Literary Journals

These journals publish essays and literary/visual pieces which can be used in teaching and accept submissions from educators and trainees who wish to publish their own creative pieces.

- *The Healing Muse* (thehealingmuse.org)
- *Ars Medica* (Mt. Sinai, Canada, www.ars-medica.ca)
- *Bellevue Literary Review* (http://www.blreview.org/)
- *Journal of General Internal Medicine ("Healing Arts" feature)*

Ars Medica consists of well-crafted, highly readable, and engaging personal narratives; essays or short stories of up to 1,500 words; and poetry of up to 100 lines. These pieces should focus on a given experience, person, or event which informs or illuminates the practice or teaching of medicine. Submissions may be written by or from the point of view of the patient, healthcare provider, family member, teacher, investigator, or trainee. If nonfiction, please either mask the subject's identity or gain their permission prior to submission.

- *Medical Humanities* (mh.bmj.com) publishes poetry
- *Health Affairs: Narrative Matters*: first-person accounts that connect to policy
- *Yale Journal for Humanities and Medicine*: prose and poetry
- *The Human Factor* (University of Missouri-Kansas City Medical School)
- Blood and Thunder (U of Oklahoma, Coll. of Medicine)
- *Pulse: Voices from the Heart of Medicine* (www.pulsemagazine.org)
- *Hospital Drive: A Journal of Reflective Practice in Word and Image* (http://hospitaldrive.med.virginia.edu/).
  "Submissions will be accepted from anyone involved with providing, teaching, studying, or researching patient care."

- *Cell 2 Soul* (www.cell2soul.org)
- *Wild Onions* (Hershey Medical Center)
- *Reflexions* (Columbia University, open to general public)
- *Plexus* (University of California, Irvine)
- *The Medical Muse* (University of New Mexico)
- *The Body Electric* (University of Illinois–Chicago College of Medicine)
- *Dermanities* (dermanties.com)
- *Hospital Drive* (http://www.hospitaldrive.med.virginia.edu/
- *JAMA*: "A Piece of My Mind."
  "Most essays published in 'A Piece of My Mind' are personal vignettes (e.g., exploring the dynamics of the patient-physician relationship) taken from wide-ranging experiences in medicine; occasional pieces express views and opinions on the myriad issues that affect the profession. If the patient(s) described in these manuscripts is identifiable, a patient permission form must be completed and signed by the patient(s) and submitted with the manuscript. Omitting data or making data less specific to de-identify patients is acceptable, but changing any such data is not acceptable. Manuscripts are not published anonymously or pseudonymously. Length limit: 1,800 words."
- *American Journal of Nursing.*
  "AJN also welcomes submissions [by nurses] of narratives, commentaries, photoessays, and other forms of writing. See specific guidelines for Reflections, Viewpoint, and some columns at http://AJN.edmgr.com or contact Editorial Director Shawn Kennedy at shawn.kennedy@wolterskluwer.com to discuss specific formats not discussed in these guidelines."
- *American Nurse Today*: nonfiction narrative and poetry by nurses.
- *Patient Education and Counseling*: "Reflective Practice."
  "The Reflective Practice section includes papers about personal or professional experiences that provide a lesson applicable to caring, humanism, and relationship in healthcare. We welcome unsolicited manuscripts. No abstract is needed. No (section) headings, no numbering. Maximum 1,500 words. First name and surname of the author and his/her institution affiliation

address, telephone and fax number and e-mail address where the corresponding author can be contacted, title of the papers and text. Submissions will be peer-reviewed by two reviewers."

- *Human Pathology*: "Pathology and the Humanities."

  "Essays, narratives, poetry, etc., on the humanistic aspects of our discipline. These narratives should be brief (2–4 typewritten pages) although the scope is less restrictive."

- *American Journal of Kidney Disease*: "In a Few Words."

  "Creative non-fiction feature. In this space, we hope to give voice to the personal experiences and stories that define kidney disease. We will accept for review nonfiction, narrative submissions up to 1,600 words, regarding the personal, ethical, or policy implications of any aspect of kidney disease in adults and children (acute kidney injury, chronic kidney disease, dialysis, transplantation, ethics, health policy, genetics, etc.). Footnotes or references are discouraged. Any submission which refers to real patients must be either unidentifiable or approved by the patient(s) described. Submissions from physicians, allied health professionals, patients, or family members are welcome. Items for consideration should be submitted via AJKD's outline manuscript handling site, www.editorialmanager.com/ajkd. Questions or requests for assistance may be directed to the editorial office staff at AJKD@tuftsmedicalcenter.org."

- *Medical Encounter* (http://www.aachonline.org/publications/medicalencounter/).

  A publication of the American Academy on Communication in Healthcare, which accepts poetry, essays, and so on about doctors and patients.

- The *American Journal of Hospice & Palliative Medicine* publishes poetry.

Journals that Publish Nonfiction Essays

- *The Lancet*
- *Academic Medicine*: "Medicine and the Arts"

  The journal's longest-running feature, this column runs on two facing pages; the left-hand page features an excerpt from literature, a poem, a photograph, etc. Literature excerpts generally run no more than 700 words and may include a very brief introduction as needed. On the right-hand page is a commentary of about 900 words that explores the relevance of the artwork to the teaching and/or practice of medicine. Since submissions cannot be fully accepted for publication until *Academic Medicine* acquires permission to reprint literary excerpts or artworks, authors should include all relevant information about the piece they are explicating (publisher, museum, dates, etc.) to enable staff editors to find and contact the copyright holder.

- *Canadian Medical Association Journal:* "Humanities" (http://www.cmaj.ca/authors/preparing.shtml)

  "The Humanities section gives readers room for reflection through reviews on books and the visual and performing arts, creative writing, photography and features on the philosophy and history of medicine. Book and arts reviews are mainly solicited by the editor. We welcome unsolicited poetry, fiction and creative nonfiction for "Room for a view" and especially value contributions that convey personal and professional experiences with a sense of immediacy and realism. The writing should be candid, but patient confidentiality must be respected. In general, prose manuscripts should be limited to 1000 words and poems to no more than 75 lines. Photography submissions are welcome, as are brief, illustrated items on unexplored corners of medical history. If you would like to be added to our list of book reviewers or would like to discuss ideas for contributions please contact the Deputy Editor, News and Humanities, Barbara Sibbald (Barbara.sibbald@cmaj.ca)."

- *Journal of General Internal Medicine:* "Text and Context"

  "Consists of excerpts from literature (novels, short stories, poetry, plays or creative non-fiction) of 200–800 words and an accompanying essay of up to 1000 words discussing the meaning of the work and linking it to the clinical or medical education literature. May include up to 3 learning objectives/discussion questions and up to 5 references, including an appropriately detailed reference of the creative work."

- *International Journal of Healthcare & Humanities* (Penn State College of Medicine, Department of Humanities; Cheryl Dellasega, PhD, editor-in-chief)
- *International Journal of the Creative Arts in Interdisciplinary Practice*
  "An international and interdisciplinary peer reviewed open access journal. Our mission is to publish, disseminate and make accessible worldwide, quality information, research and knowledge about the creative arts in health and interdisciplinary practice."
- *Annals of Internal Medicine*: "Medical Writings"
- *Journal of Medical Humanities*
- *Literature and Medicine*
- *Medical Humanities*
- *The Pharos*
- *Yale Journal for Humanities in Medicine*
- *Atrium* (www.bioethics.northwestern.edu/atrium/index.html)
- *International Journal of the Creative Arts in Interdisciplinary Practice* (http://www.ijcaip.com/)
- *Philosophy, Ethics, and Humanities in Medicine* (www.peh-med.com)
- *Perspectives in Biology and Medicine*
- *Patient Education and Counseling*
- *Medical Education*
- *Journal for Learning through the Arts*
  This is an exclusively e-journal, published by e-Scholarship University of California. It is a peer-reviewed journal published once a year. While its focus is primarily on use of the arts in K-12 education, it includes a regular section on "Literature and the Arts in Medical Education," which includes one or two articles.
- *Hektoen International: A Journal of Medical Humanities* (http://www.hektoeninternational.org/Journal_submission.htm)
  - Articles on art, anthropology, ethics, literature, healthcare, history, and humanities as related to medicine. It also maintains an art gallery and an online library for storing articles and reprints.

Journals that Publish Student Writing

- *Journal of General Internal Medicine*'s Annual Creative Medical Writing Contest
- *Dermanities* (dermanities.com)
- *Body Electric* (University of Illinois)
- *The Legible Script,* a national literary journal (http://thelegiblescript.org/)
  "We are seeking talent in the areas of prose (to include essays and short fiction), poetry, personal statements and art/photography."
- *Personae* (Northwestern University)
- *Veritas* (University of Virginia; http://www.student.virginia.edu/~veritas/)
- MS*JAMA* (http://jama.ama-assn.org/ms_current.dtl)
  Submit creative writing to: Teri Reynolds treynol@itsa.ucsf.edu or Teri.Reynolds@ucsf.edu
- *The Healer's Voice* (American Medical Student Association; http://www.amsa.org/humed/hv/)
  "Our national online monthly creative expression journal: healers_voice@amsa.org"
- *Iris* (University of North Carolina journal of medicine, literature, and visual art; UNC Medical and Chapel Hill community only)
- *Connective Tissue* (for University of Texas-Galveston med students)

Chapter 2: Redirecting the Clinical Gaze: Film as a Tool of Critical Reflection in Residency Training

Suggested Reading

Alexander, Matthew, Lenahan, Patricia, and Pavlov, Anna, eds. *Cinemeducation: A Comprehensive Guide to Using Film in Medical Education*. Boca Raton, FL: CRC Press; 1999.

Alexander, Matthew, Lenahan, Patricia, and Pavlov, Anna, eds. *Cinemeducation: Using Film and Other Visual Media in Graduate and Medical Education*. Boca Raton, FL: CRC Press; 2012.

Bordwell, David, and Thompson, Kristin. *Film Art: An Introduction,* 10th ed. New York: McGraw-Hill Education; 2012.

Cartwright, Lisa. *Screening the Body: Tracing Medicine's Visual Culture.* Minneapolis: University of Minnesota Press; 1995.

Colt, Henri, Quadrelli, Silvia, and Friedman, Lester. eds. *The Picture of Health: Medical Ethics and the Movies.* New York: Oxford University Press; 2011.

Glasser, Brian. *Medicinema: Doctors in Film.* Boca Raton, FL: CRC Press; 2010.

Wedding, Danny, Boyd, Mary Ann, and Niemiec, Ryan M., eds. *Movies and Mental Illness: Using Films to Understand Psychopathology.* Boston: Hogrefe & Huber; 2005.

Jones, Therese, Wear, Delese, and Friedman, Lester D., eds. *Health Humanities Reader.* New Brunswick, NJ: Rutgers University Press; 2014.

Nichols, Bill. *Representing Reality: Issues and Concepts in Documentary.* Bloomington: Indiana University Press; 1992.

Ostherr, Kirsten. *Medical Visions: Producing the Patient Through Film, Television, and Imaging.* New York: Oxford University Press; 2013.

Reagan, Leslie J., Tomes, Nancy, and Treichler, Paula A. eds. *Medicine's Moving Pictures: Medicine, Health, and Bodies in American Film and Television.* Rochester, NY: University of Rochester Press; 2007.

Sobchack, Vivian. Inscribing ethical space: Ten propositions on death, representation, and documentary. *Q Rev Film Video.* 1984;9:4:283–300.

Sontag, Susan. *Illness as Metaphor.* New York: Farrar, Straus, and Giroux; 1978.

Films

Triage: Dr. James Orbinski's Humanitarian Dilemma. Patrick Reed; 2008.
Themes: global health, health equity, community engagement, personal reflection, advocacy, trauma, bearing witness, documentary
Kids. Larry Clark; 1995.
Themes: adolescent medicine, sexual health, substance abuse, group dynamics
The Necessities of Life. Benoît Pilon; 2008.
Themes: aboriginal health, cross-cultural healthcare, patient/client-physician relationships, communication
Cléo from 5 to 7. Agnès Varda; 1962.

Themes: illness narratives (cancer), uncertainty, mortality, gender, meaning

Frankenstein. James Whale; 1931.

Themes: research ethics, historical representations of researchers/ physicians, modernity and progress narratives

Warrendale. Allan King; 1967.

Themes: child psychiatry, residential treatment, institutions, *cinéma vérité*, documentary ethics, treatment controversy

Blue. Derek Jarman; 1993.

Themes: patient/client experience, end of life, AIDS, formal experimentation

Away from Her. Sarah Polley; 2006.

Themes: aging and the caregiver perspective, Alzheimer's disease

The Thing. John Carpenter; 1982.

Themes: body horror as social commentary (HIV/AIDS), contagion and group dynamics

The Elephant Man. David Lynch; 1980.

Themes: power and the patient/client-physician relationship, the clinical gaze, exploitation

For lesson plans, see http://cahh.ca/resources/ouplesson-plans/

Chapter 3: Narrative Medicine in Postgraduate Medical Education: Practices, Principles, Paradoxes

Suggested Reading

Charon R. *Narrative Medicine: Honoring the Stories of Illness.* New York: Oxford University Press; 2008.

Charon R, DasGupta S, Hermann N, et al. *The Principles and Practice of Narrative Medicine.* New York: Oxford University Press; 2016.

Greenhalgh T, Hurwitz B. Why study narrative? *BMJ.* 1999;318 (7175):48–50.

For Other Approaches to Reflective Writing

Peterkin, Allan D. *Portfolio to Go: 1000+ Reflective Writing Prompts and Provocations.* Toronto: University of Toronto Press; 2016.

Workshops and Diploma Training

http://www.narrativepractice.org (a not-for-profit training center in Boston)

http://www.narrativemedicine.org (Columbia University, New York)

http://www.mountsinai.on.ca/care/psych/staff-education-programs/ mspi (University of Toronto Narrative Atelier)

For lesson plans, see http://cahh.ca/resources/ouplesson-plans/

Chapter 4: Bioethics

Suggested Reading

Beauchamp T, Childress J. *Principles of Biomedical Ethics*, 7th ed. London: Oxford University Press; 2012. http://www.oupcanada. com/catalog/9780199924585.html

Ferreres A, Angelos P, Singer E, eds. *Ethical Issues in Surgical Care*. Chicago: American College of Surgeons; 2017. https://www. facs.org/education/division-of-education/publications/ ethical-issues-in-surgical-care

Hébert P. *Doing Right: A Practical Guide to Ethics for Physicians and Medical Trainees*, 3rd ed. Toronto: Oxford University Press; 2014. http://www.oupcanada.com/catalog/9780199005529.html

Hébert P. *Good Medicine: The Art of Ethical Care*. Toronto: Random House; 2016. https://www.goodreads.com/book/show/ 25982584-good-medicine

Sadler J, Van Staden W, Fulford K, eds. *Oxford Handbook of Psychiatric Ethics*. Oxford: Oxford University Press; 2015. https://global.oup. com/academic/product/oxford-handbook-of-psychiatric-ethics-9780199663880?cc=ca&lang=en&

Web Resources

Recommended Curriculum Guidelines for Family Medicine Residents: Medical Ethics. American Academy of Family Physicians. http://www.aafp.org/dam/AAFP/documents/medical_education_ residency/program_directors/Reprint279_Ethics.pdf

Royal College of General Practitioners of UK Curriculum Statement. 3.3 Clinical Ethics and Values-Based Practice. http://www.gmc-uk.org/3_3_Ethics_2006_01.pdf_30448781.pdf

Ethics in Family Medicine: Faculty Handbook. College of Family
Physicians of Canada. October 2012. http://www.cfpc.ca/
uploadedFiles/Resources/Resource_Items/Health_Professionals/
Faculty%20Handbook_Edited_FINAL_05Nov12.pdf

Royal College of Canada. Bioethics. Curriculum. http://www.
royalcollege.ca/rcsite/bioethics-e

Royal Australiasian College of Physicians. Resources. https://www.
racp.edu.au/fellows/resources/curated-collections/ethics

For lesson plans, see http://cahh.ca/resources/ouplesson-plans/

APPENDIX I. Six medical competencies. Adapted from the ACGME
outcomes project.

Chapter 5: The Visible Curriculum

Sample Collections of Visual Art for Use in Medical Education

Art and Images in Psychiatry: JAMA's searchable database of historical/contemporary artworks and associated essays which explore aspects of mental illness: http://jamanetwork.com/collections/6261/art-and-images-in-psychiatry

NYU's database of searchable, annotated material, including paintings, photographs, and sculpture: http://medhum.med.nyu.edu

Bordin, Georgio, and Laura Polo D'Ambrosio. 2010. *Medicine in Art.* Trans. Jay Hyams. Los Angeles: J. Paul Getty Museum.

Out of Our Heads: University of Bristol Medical Humanities program's online searchable gallery of visual and written art: www.outofourheads.net/oooh/handler.php?p=homepage

Sample Course Materials

Yale's online example of the use of narrative painting to strengthen visual literacy in dermatology, including discussion points, grading key, grading sheet, and examples of artwork used: https://medicine.yale.edu/dermatology/education/obvski

Visual Learning website (Brighton University): Drawing subsection: http://about.brighton.ac.uk/visuallearning/drawing/

In addition to links to other resources on drawing in education, this site houses downloadable PDFs of the "Drawing to Learn: Visual Learning in Higher Education" booklets by Pauline Ridley and Angela Rogers. This series includes a booklet devoted to "Clinical Education, Health and Social Care" which contains suggestions for drawing exercises tailored for diverse types of learning objectives.

Sample Videos about Learning to Look in the Galleries

A collaboration between the Yale School of Medicine and the Yale Center for British Art: https://www.youtube.com/watch?v=oL1b1tMNI4E

Part of the Arts and Humanities Initiative at Harvard Medical School: https://www.youtube.com/watch?v=emuj7Sp24dw

Video recording on the collaboration between art museums and medical schools, from the Edith O'Donnell Institute of Art History at the University of Texas at Dallas: https://www.utdallas.edu/arthistory/medicine/moma-2016/video/index.html

Sites that Explore Visual Literacy

- Visual Thinking Strategies: vtshome.org
- *Arts Practica*: medical education consultancy: www.artspractica.com
- Insight Institute: an educational non-profit that uses the arts to develop better observation and communication skills: www.insightinstitute.org
- Toledo Museum of Art: visual literacy resources: http://www.toledomuseum.org/learn/visual-literacy

Sample Learner Exhibits

University of Michigan Medical School, Family Centered Experience, examples of Interpretive Projects: www.med.umich.edu/lrc/fce/

The Body Electric, a juried digital art exhibit in conjunction with the International Conference on Residency Education: https://thebodyelectric-lecorpselectrique.ca/

White Coat/Warm Art, a juried digital/live art exhibit in conjunction with the Canadian Conference on Medical Education: www.mededconference.ca/meetings-and-events/white-coat-warm-heart

Synesthesia, an annual art show organized by University of Toronto Faculty of Medicine and ArtBeat, its student health humanities blog: health-humanities.com/invitation-to-participate-in-synesthesia-2017/

Selected Works of Graphic Medicine (Comics)

Graphic Medicine website: http://www.graphicmedicine.org/, a continuously updated clearinghouse for all things graphic medicine related.

- Fies B. *Mom's Cancer*. Harry N. Abrams; 2006.
- Czerwiec MK. *Taking Turns: Stories from HIV/AIDS Care Unit 371*. Pennsylvania State University Press; 2017.

- Williams I. *The Bad Doctor*. Myriad Editions; 2014.
- Small D. *Stitches: A Memoir*. W.W. Norton; 2009.
- Forney E. *Marbles: Mania, Depression, Michelangelo, and Me*. Gotham Books; 2012.

For lesson plans, see http://cahh.ca/resources/ouplesson-plans/

Chapter 6: Teaching the Social Sciences in Residency

Sample Teaching Materials Incorporating Behavioral and Social Sciences (BSS) Skills and Social Determinants of Health (SDOH) Content

Enhancing Behavioral and Social Science at the Bedside: Core Skills for Clinicians and Teachers. https://www.mededportal.org/publication/10032 29 – A 120-minute faculty-training workshop

The SBS Toolbox: Clinical Pearls from the Social and Behavioral Sciences. https://www.mededportal.org/publication/7980 30. A curricular resource summarizing key BSS topics.

Exploring Health Systems Within the Context of Social Determinants of Health: A Global Health Case Study. https://www.mededportal.org/publication/10457 36. A case study centered on SDOH content.

From Identification to Advocacy: A Module for Teaching Social Determinants of Health. https://www.mededportal.org/publication/10266 37. A multipart curriculum centered on applying SDOH to individual- and system-level advocacy activities.

Further Reading

Bromley E, Braslow JT. Teaching critical thinking in psychiatric training: A role for the social sciences. *Am J Psychiatry*. 2008; 165(11):1396–401. doi:10.1176/appi.ajp.2008.08050690

Charon R, Holmboe E, Holmes JH, et al. Behavioral and Social Science Foundations for Future Physicians: Report of the Behavioral and Social Science Expert Panel. https://www.aamc.org/download/271020/data/behavioralandsocialsciencefoundationsforfuturephysicians

Cuff PA, Vanselow N. *Improving Medical Education: Enhancing the Behavioral and Social Science Content of Medical School Curricula.* Washington, DC: National Academies Press, 2004.

Croft D, Jay SJ, Meslin EM, Gaffney MM, Odell JD. Perspective: Is it time for advocacy training in medical education? *Acad Med.* 2012; 87(9):1165–1170.

Daniels AH, Bariteau JT, Grabel Z, DiGiovanni CW. Prospective analysis of a novel orthopedic residency advocacy education program. *R I Med J.* 2014; 97(10):43–46.

Hothersall EJ. Project update: Assessing the behavioural and social science curricula components for undergraduate medical students: A BEME systematic review. http://bemecollaboration. org/downloads/2658/Project%20Update%20August%20 2016.pdf.

Martin D, Hum S, Han M, Whitehead C. Laying the foundation: Teaching policy and advocacy to medical trainees. *Med Teach.* 2013; 35(5): 352–358.

For lesson plans, see http://cahh.ca/resources/ouplesson-plans/

Chapter 7: The Use of Theatre with Medical Residents: An Embodied Approach to Learning about Self and Other

Resources

The following resources are useful to those who wish to develop new seminars and workshops but may not have training in teaching theater/performance and for those who would like to more deeply understand various approaches to theater, performance, and theater as research. They are texts from the Western performance canon that are specifically useful to performance-based teaching and learning for non-theater professionals (like doctors) and that relate to the elements and methods of theater practice included in the chapter.

Alda, Alan. *If I Understood You, Would I Have This Look on My Face? My Adventures in the Art and Science of Relating and Communicating.* New York: Random House, 2017. Detailed description of work using improvisation to assist scientists in communication.

Boal, Augusto. *Theatre of the Oppressed*. 3rd ed. New York: Pluto Press, 2000. Describes the theory upon which Boal's methods are based.

Boal, Augusto. *Games for Actors and Non-Actors*. New York: Routledge, 2002. Performance-based exercises and games.

Improv Encyclopedia. http://improvencyclopedia.org/. Exercises, warm-ups, resources, games, and glossary organized by specific skills.

Johnstone, Keith. *Impro: Improvisation and the Theatre*. New York: Routledge, 2012. Seminal text on improvisation for the theater.

Kemp, Rick. *Embodied Acting: What Neuroscience Tells Us About Performance*. New York: Routledge, 2012. An excellent source-book for understanding the physical and cognitive mechanisms at play in performance. Includes exercises from master teachers and provides scientific justification for the use of theater which may be helpful to secure funding.

Norris, Joe. *Playbuilding as Qualitative Research: A Participatory Arts-Based Approach*. New York: Routledge, 2016. A rich source for researchers who wish to use theater as a form of research and artists who are interested in research-inspired work. Provides a common language for researchers and artists.

Rodenburg, Patsy. *The Second Circle: How to Use Positive Energy for Success in Every Situation*. New York: W. W. Norton, 2012. Used in theater conservatories as a source to learn awareness of how interpersonal energy affects performance, communication, and relationships.

Smith, Hazel, and Dean, Roger. *Practice Led Research, Research Led Practice in the Creative Arts*. Edinburgh, UK: University of Edinburgh Press, 2011. Source for thinking about methodologies used in creative practices as research.

Spolin, Viola. *Improvisation for the Theatre*. Evanston, IL: Northwestern University Press, 1999. Exercises with expert guidance on in-the-moment coaching of learners/actors.

Reader's Theater Possibilities

The following plays and texts with themes of illness may be useful for Reader's Theater seminars for residents:

Chekhov, Anton. *The Seagull*
Chekhov, Anton. *Uncle Vanya*

Edson, Margaret. *Wit*
Flacks, Diane. *The Waiting Room*
Kramer, Larry. *The Normal Heart*
Kane, Sarah. *Psychosis 4.48*
Kushner, Tony. *Angels in America*
Letts, Tracy. *August Osage County*
Oyebode, Femi. *Madness at the Theatre*
Weiss, Peter. *The Marat Sade*

For lesson plans, see http://cahh.ca/resources/ouplesson-plans/

Chapter 8: Promoting Collaborative Competencies: Using the Arts and the Humanities to Enhance Relational Practice and Teamwork

Suggested Reading

D'Amour D, Oandasan I. Interprofessionality as the field of interprofessional practice and interprofessional education: An emerging concept. *J Interprof Care*. 2005; 19(Suppl 1): 8–20.

Hall P, Brajman S, Weaver L, Grassau P, Varpio L. Learning collaborative teamwork: An argument for incorporating the humanities. *J Interprof Care*. 2014; 28(6): 519–525. doi: 10.3109/13561820.2014.915513

Lie D, Forest C, Kysh L, Sinclair, L. Interprofessional education and practice guide no. 5: Interprofessional teaching for prequalification students in clinical settings. *J Interprof Care*. 2016; 30(3): 324–330. doi:10.3109/13561820.2016.1141752

Sargeant J, Hill T, Breau L. Development and testing of a scale to assess interprofessional education (IPE) facilitation skills. *J Contin Educ Health Prof*. 2010; 30(2): 126–131. doi: 10.1002/chp.20069

Willgerodtl M, Abu-Rish Blakeney E, Brock D, Liner D, Murphy N, Zierler B. Interprofessional education and practice guide no. 4: Developing and sustaining interprofessional education at an academic health center. *J Interprof Care*. 2015;29(5): 421–425. doi: 10.3109/13561820.2015.1039117

For lesson plans, see http://cahh.ca/resources/ouplesson-plans/

Chapter 9: Teaching History of Medicine/Healthcare in Residency

Sources in the History of Medicine

We realize that residents curious about history are not mainly setting themselves up for careers as research scholars. So this historical guide leans more toward faculty members who might enjoy bringing history to residents, as opposed to outfitting residents to enter the archives. Yet in history, the reading of the secondary literature is often narrowly interblended with research in primary sources. This is the charm of the subject! So the following paragraphs address both the classroom teachers of medical history and the eager researchers.

The standard bibliographic index to medical literature has been the so-called "IndexCat": the online *Index-Catalogue of the Library of the Surgeon-General's Office,* printed from 1880 to 1961 in five series consisting of 61 volumes containing almost 4 million books and articles, available online at http://indexcat.nlm.nih.gov. Its successors are the *Index Medicus* and the online PubMed. But, unlike these later indexes, the "Surgeon-General's Catalogue," as it is called, also includes books. For anyone contemplating original research in the history of medicine, this would be the starting point. An essential guide to "priorities," or first descriptions of something, and to seminal works in the primary literature, is Leslie T. Morton, *Garrison and Morton: A Medical Bibliography,* 5th ed. (London: Gower, 1991). (An updated version went online in 2015 as *Morton's Medical Bibliography,* 5th ed.)

Online Resources

Due to the diligence of energetic and computer-literate younger scholars, we now have two major indexes of sources and resources in the history of medicine. The Society for the Social History of Medicine has compiled an extensive review of activities in the UK (and elsewhere) at https://sshm.org/links. As well, the History of Medicine Program at McMaster University in Hamilton, Ontario, has assembled lists of digitized archival materials and blogs across the entire range of the history of medicine and science: the History of Medicine and Medical Humanities Research Web Portal.

Key Journals

History of medicine content sometimes appears in biomedical journals, but a richer source are more specialized journals:

- *Academic Medicine.* 1926–present. Official peer-reviewed journal of the Association of American Medical Colleges. Began July 1926 as its *Bulletin*; 1929–1951: *Journal*; 1951–1988: *Journal of Medical Education.* Present title adopted 1989.
- *Bulletin of the History of Medicine.* Baltimore, MD: Johns Hopkins University Press. 1933–present. Official organ of both the American Association for the History of Medicine and the Institute of the History of Medicine at Johns Hopkins University.
- *Canadian Bulletin of Medical History/Bulletin canadien d'histoire de la médecine.* Toronto: University of Toronto Press, 1984–present. Official publication of the Canadian Society for the History of Medicine/Société canadienne d'histoire de la médecine.
- *Journal of the History of Medicine and Allied Sciences.* Oxford University Press, 1946–present.
- *Medical Humanities.* Institute of Medical Ethics (IME) London: BMJ Publishing Group. 2000–present. Inaugural issue 26(1) June 2000. Launched as a companion to the IME's *Journal of Medical Ethics*, 26(3) Feb. 2000; see Gillon, Ranaan, "Welcome to medical humanities—and why" (Editorial): http://jme.bmj.com/content/26/3/155.
- *Journal of the Medical Library Association.* Chicago: Medical Library Association, 2002–present. Began in 1898 as *Medical Libraries*; 1903–1907: *Medical Library and Historical Journal*; 1911–2001: *Bulletin of the Medical Library Association.* Baltimore: Johns Hopkins Press.
- *Hektoen International: A Journal of Medical Humanities. Chicago: Hektoen Institute of Medicine. 2008–Present.*

It is thus evident that the history of medicine represents a deep scholarly stream flowing through the heart of medical humanities. Studying medical history may make you not only a better physician; it may give you an exciting and lifelong cultural pursuit.

For lesson plans, see http://cahh.ca/resources/ouplesson-plans/

Chapter 10: Difficult Conversations: Evaluating the Medical Humanities

Suggested Qualitative Research Readings

Carter SM, Little M. Justifying knowledge, justifying method, taking action: Epistemologies, methodologies, and methods in qualitative research. *Qual Health Res.* 2007;17(10):1316–1328.

Haynes K. Reflexivity in qualitative research. In: Symon G, Cassell C, eds. *Qualitative Organizational Research: Core Methods and Current Challenges*. London: SAGE; 2012: 72–89.

Ng S, et al. Qualitative research in medical education: Methodologies and methods. In: Swanwic T, ed. *Understanding Medical Education: Evidence, Theory and Practice*. Chichester, UK: John Wiley; 2013: 371–384.

Lingard L, et al. Grounded theory, mixed methods, and action research. *BMJ.* 2008;337:567.

Starks H, Trinidad SB. Choose your method: A comparison of phenomenology, discourse analysis, and grounded theory. *Qual Health Res.* 2007;17(10):1372–1380.

Suggested Readings on Research Method in Medical Education

Barone T, Eisner EW. *Arts Based Research*. London: SAGE; 2011.

Chilton G, Leavy P. Arts-based research practice: merging social research and the creative arts. In: *The Oxford Handbook of Qualitative Research*. New York: Oxford University Press; 2014:403–422.

Knowles JG, Cole AL. *Handbook of the Arts in Qualitative Research: Perspectives, Methodologies, Examples, and Issues*. London: SAGE; 2008.

Glasby J, Walshe K, Harvey G. What counts as "evidence" in "evidence-based practice"? *Evid Policy.* 2007;3(3):325–327.

Joseph K, Bader K, Wilson S, Walker M, Stephens M, Varpio L. Unmasking identity dissonance: exploring medical students' professional identity formation through mask making. *Perspect Med Educ.* 2017;6(2):99–107.

Green MJ. Comics and medicine: peering into the process of professional identity formation. *Acad Med.* 2015;90(6):774–779.

Shapiro D, Tomasa L, Koff NA. Patients as teachers, medical students as filmmakers: the video slam, a pilot study. *Acad Med*. 2009;84(9): 1235–1243.

Kelly M, Bennett D, O'Flynn S, Foley T. A picture tells 1000 words: learning teamwork in primary care. *Clin Teach*. 2013;10(2): 113–117.

Gilligan C, Spencer R, Weinberg MK, Bertsch T. On the listening guide. In: Hesse-Biber SN, Leavy P, eds. *Emergent Methods in Social Research*. London: SAGE; 2006:253–268.

Kress GR, Van Leeuwen T. *Reading Images: The Grammar of Visual Design*. New York: Psychology Press; 1996.

Gardner H. *The Unschooled Mind: How Children Think and How Schools Should Teach*. New York: Basic Books; 2011.

Wang CC, Pies CA. Family, maternal, and child health through photovoice. *Matern Child Health J*. 2004;8(2):95–102.

Rose G. *Visual Methodologies: An Introduction to Researching with Visual Materials*. London: SAGE; 2016.

Lorenz KA, Steckart MJ, Rosenfeld KE. End-of-life education using the dramatic arts: the Wit educational initiative. *Acad Med*. 2004;79(5):481–486.

Brett-MacLean P, Yiu V, Farooq A. Exploring professionalism in undergraduate medical and dental education through forum theatre. *J Learn Arts*. 2012;8(1):n1.

Thelwall M, Delgado MM. Arts and humanities research evaluation: no metrics please, just data. *J Document*. 2015;71(4):817–833.

Trautmann J. *Healing Arts in Dialogue: Medicine and Literature*. Carbondale: Southern Illinois University Press ;1981.

Von Bertalanffy L. The history and status of general systems theory. *Acad Manage J*. 1972;15(4):407–426.

Ringsted C, Hodges B, Scherpbier A. The research compass: An introduction to research in medical education: AMEE Guide No. 56. *Med Teach*. 2011;33(9):695–709.

Watling CJ, Lingard L. Grounded theory in medical education research: AMEE Guide No. 70. *Med Teach*. 2012;34(10): 850–861.

Coverdale JH, et al. Writing for academia: Getting your research into print: AMEE Guide No. 74. *Med Teach*. 2013;35(2):e926–e934.

Tavakol M, Sandars J. Quantitative and qualitative methods in medical education research: AMEE Guide No 90: Part I. *Med Teach.* 2014;36(9):746–756.

Tavakol M, Sandars J. Quantitative and qualitative methods in medical education research: AMEE Guide No 90: Part II. *Med Teach.* 2014;36(10):838–848.

Dennick R. Twelve tips for incorporating educational theory into teaching practices. *Med Teach.* 2012;34(8):618–624. cvefr

Turner TL, et al. Methodologies and study designs relevant to medical education research. *Int Rev Psychiatry.* 2013;25(3):301–310.

For lesson plans, see http://cahh.ca/resources/ouplesson-plans/

Chapter 11: How to Fund and Promote Arts-Based Initiatives in Postgraduate Medical Education

There are great many places you can apply to for funding of your Medical Humanities initiatives. The Grantspace FQA helps you categorize your funding requests: http://grantspace.org/tools/knowledge-base

Once you have figured out what type of grant you are applying for, see the following sampling of US, Canada, and UK funding sources that may be of interest to you Just bear in mind that criteria change from time to time and deadlines for applications are a crucial element.

Suggested Reading

The Grants Register 2016: The Complete Guide to Postgraduate Funding Worldwide. New York: Palgrave Macmillan.

To navigate the treacherous waters of the Pharma industry sponsorship, you should consult this website: http://www.nofreelunch.org/

In the United States:
https://www.neh.gov/
http://www.gold-foundation.org/resources/
https://dsp.research.uiowa.edu/private-funding-arts-humanities
https://www.arts.gov

http://macyfoundation.org
http://www.johnahartford.org
http://www.greenwall.org
http://www.humanities.ufl.edu/funding-other.html

In the UK:
https://wellcome.ac.uk/what-we-do/teams/humanities-and-social-science-team
http://www.britac.ac.uk/funding-opportunities
http://torch.ox.ac.uk/medical-humanities-programme-grants
http://www.ahrc.ac.uk
http://www.phil.cam.ac.uk/research/research-opps/ahshss-booklet-july2013.pdf

In Canada:
http://medhumanities.mcmaster.ca/index/grants-for-student-research
http://healtharts.ca/category/links/
http://www.nshrf.ca/hostedfunding
http://www.sshrc-crsh.gc.ca/funding-financement/index-eng.aspx
http://www.ams-inc.on.ca/funding-opportunities/
http://canuckhm.ca/considering-funding-part-iii-cihr-and-the-medical-humanities/?doing_wp_cron=1490536730.3383901119232177734375
http://www.science.gc.ca/eic/site/063.nsf/eng/h_FEE7261A.html?OpenDocument

Index

Tables, figures, and boxes are indicated by an italic *t*, *f*, and *b* following the page number.